ARCHIVING MEDICAL VIOLENCE

Archiving Medical Violence

Consent and the Carceral State

CHRISTOPHER PERREIRA

University of Minnesota Press
Minneapolis
London

The University of Minnesota Press gratefully acknowledges the financial assistance provided for the publication of this book by the Department of Ethnic Studies and the Office of Research Affairs at UC San Diego.

Portions of chapter one are adapted from "'Suppose for a Moment, That Keanu Had Reasoned Thus': Contagious Debts and Prisoner-Patient Consent in Nineteenth-Century Hawai'i," *Journal of Transnational American Studies* 8, no. 1 (2017), https://doi.org/10.5070/T881023860. Chapter 3 was originally published as "Consumed by Disease: Medical Archives, Latino Fictions, and Carceral Health Imaginaries," in *Captivating Technology: Race, Carceral Technoscience, and Liberatory Imagination in Everyday Life*, ed. Ruha Benjamin, 50–66; copyright 2019 Duke University Press. All rights reserved. Reprinted by permission of the publisher, www.dukeupress.edu.

Published by the University of Minnesota Press
111 Third Avenue South, Suite 290
Minneapolis, MN 55401-2520
http://www.upress.umn.edu

ISBN 978-1-5179-0711-2 (hc)
ISBN 978-1-5179-0712-9 (pb)

A Cataloging-in-Publication record for this book is available from the Library of Congress.

CONTENTS

PREFACE AND ACKNOWLEDGMENTS

For many people writing, thinking, and teaching about histories and legacies of racism, the Covid-19 pandemic put into focus the immediacy of that work for understanding this moment. The *Los Angeles Review of Books*, for example, published a collection of short essays in April 2020 called, perhaps uncomfortably, *The Quarantine Files: Thinkers in Self-Isolation*, only months after shutdowns began. In that collection is a piece by Saidiya Hartman titled "The Death Toll," in which, in five paragraphs, she masterfully locates the meaning of the pandemic in the history of enslavement and colonialism—a train of thought she notes was prompted by the routine act of preparing for her seminar. Stuck on a single sentence from Tiffany Lethabo King's *The Black Shoals: Offshore Formations of Black and Native Studies*—"Everyday life is marked by grotesque interludes with Black and Indigenous death in the streets or in the plains"—and aware that several of her students were mourning the losses of loved ones, early deaths caused by this new coronavirus, Hartman pauses to take stock of the sizable issue underlying the warlike campaign that medical discourse was then trying to work out. "How does one navigate across [these] scales of death?"[1] What is this unfixed yet tethered *thing*, Hartman asks, pulling and tugging, between the "everyday character of catastrophe, the uneventfulness of black and Indigenous death," and the recent havoc and devastation made visible by this pandemic? Turning to the *New England Journal of Medicine*, where medical knowledge has spoken and archived itself for centuries, provides unsettling answers for Hartman. The United States is surely going to face similar shortages of ventilators and health-care worker protections as in Italy, the authors of the journal article note, but with more devastating consequences. As the virus spreads across the country, and as waves of patients fill the hospitals, should we not be asking about the fundamentally basic question in front of us: How will doctors decide who gets a ventilator, who on the medical staff gets personal protection equipment (PPE), and who does not? "No matter which estimate we use, there are not enough ventilators for patients with Covid-19 in the upcoming months," the authors of the *New England Journal of Medicine* article write. "Equally worrisome is the lack of adequate PPE for frontline health care workers, including respirators, gloves, face shields, gowns, and hand sanitizer. In Italy, health care workers experienced high rates of infection and death partly because of inadequate access to PPE. And recent estimates here in the United States suggest that we will need far more respirators and surgical masks than are currently available."[2] The authors raise the concern, warn of the coming devastation, but do little more than this, perhaps because answering the question of who lives and who dies imagines a road to inaction rather than the immediate and practical conditions for practicing medicine that are needed. But Hartman, whose writing is keenly attuned to the ways the production of archival knowledge is tethered to white supremacy and racial capitalism, is willing to speculate about this question "the doctors prefer to avoid."

> Triage is the response to the crisis, a crisis exacerbated in the United States by the 'no state' state and capitalism, by racism and white nationalism, by lies and more lies, by mismanagement, by opting for death, by the lack of universal health care. . . . Medicine has a pernicious history of racism and ableism. Even when hospitals are not overtaxed and equipment is not in short supply, I am not a priority. As empirical studies document again and again, the health-care system is routinely indifferent to black suffering, doubting the shared sentience of bodies in pain, uncertain if the human is an expansive category or an exclusive one, if indeed a human is perceived at all. Who lives and who dies? I fear the answer to such a question. I think I know what it is.

Archiving Medical Violence asks questions about who lives and who dies, not only in the triage of pandemics but in the mundane acts of medical experimentation, quarantine, incarceration, and other spaces and narratives that situate nonwhite racialized bodies as usable to forward medical knowledge and to classify it as progress—what I have termed in this book *medical violence*. Two years have passed since the start of the Covid-19 pandemic, and as I finish this manuscript over six million deaths have been recorded globally, according to the World Health Organization.[3] While many continue to grieve and navigate personal and community losses, at the level of national narrative there is little sense that a collective grieving has occurred, or even begun. How does our frame shift when we consider the death toll as both a horror on its own and, at the same time, part of a continuum within racial capitalism—as part of a process of navigating the "scales of death"? As connected to the management and mismanagement of governments, public health leaders, and institutions responding to the virus, and at the same time as a racial logic that structures the very questions and language with which to name these phenomena? This is, of course, more than any book can attempt to answer. In fact, as I tried I felt language's limitations at every turn. Yet these questions permeate—perhaps *haunt* is the better word—all the different ways into knowing what it is we say we know about how to navigate this current moment.

I began asking questions that resist easy answers long before I found a language that could accommodate the contradictions that I believed made up the world around me. For that, I need to first thank my parents, who taught me (without "teaching") so many things. From you I learned what it means to face struggle with kindness and generosity. I want to thank you for all the ways you modeled love and tenderness, especially when I could not understand that is what you were doing. When I started community college in the late nineties, I had no idea how much it would shape the kinds of questions I would later pursue for years to come. Those classrooms were unexpectedly important spaces for me to start seeing incarceration and criminalization as the unnatural thing that it is. This was one start to the project that became this book, and at the same time did not become this book. I cannot begin to thank the many people who created even the smallest spaces for those ideas, questions, and contradictions. I want to express my deepest thanks to those who guided me during my dissertation work, when those questions were underpinning all of it, while I was a graduate student in the Department of Literature at UC San Diego. I was and still am grateful for the lessons learned with my committee—Dennis Childs, Lisa Lowe, Curtis Marez, Rosaura Sánchez, and Shelley Streeby—who were much more than teachers (though they were also incredible teachers) and always friends who modeled ways to do political work in and beyond academia. Thanks to all the folks involved with Students Against Mass Incarceration at UCSD, Californians United for a Responsible Budget, All of Us or None, and San Diego No More Prisons. I am grateful to many others in the Literature Department who were generous with their time and knowledge, including Sara Johnson, Luis Martín-Cabrera, Fatima El-Tayeb, Beatrice Pita, Meg Wesling, Jorge Mariscal, Stephanie Jed, and Don Wayne.

I thank my colleagues in the Department of American Studies at the University of Kansas for taking me in as their colleague. They made room and did not hold it against me when I fumbled through the job. I need to thank Ben Chappell, Elizabeth Esch, Nishani Frazier, Jennifer Hamer, Nicole Hodges Persley, Margaret Kelley, Joo Ok Kim, Clarence Lang, Cheryl Lester, Valerie Mendoza, Ray Mizumura-Pence, Terri Rockhold, David Roediger, Sherrie Tucker, and Robert Warrior. Special thanks to Cécile Accilien, Zahir Mikah Accilien, Giselle Anatol, Hannah Bailey, José Héctor Cadena, Ignacio Carvajal, Lydia Epp Schmidt, Nate Freiburger, Maryemma Graham, Neill Kennedy, Margarita Nuñez Arroyo, Marilyn Ortega, Najarian Peters, Magalí Rabasa, Imani Wadud, and Omaris Zamora. The Department of Ethnic Studies at UC San Diego welcomed me, and I am thrilled to have them as colleagues, co-conspirators, friends, and comrades. My thanks to Patrick Anderson, Yen Le Espiritu, Ross Frank, José Fusté, Andrew Jolivétte, Curtis Marez, Kianna Middleton, Holly Okonkwo, Shaista Patel, Roy Pérez, Christen Sasaki, Shelley Streeby, Daphne Taylor-García, and K. Wayne Yang. My gratitude goes to the administrative team in Ethnic Studies: Christa Ludeking, Cecilia Ozkan, Mónica Rodriquez de Cabaza, and Amanda Vassall. For your work, your time, your care, and your person, I wish to thank Cécile Accilien, Andrew Amoral, Maile Arvin, Aimee Bahng, Crystal Baik, Benjamin Balthaser, Ruha Benjamin, Victor Betts, Julie Burelle, José Héctor Cadena, Juvenal Caporale, Ignacio Carvajal, Bianet Castellanos, Susy Chávez, Dennis Childs, Saranella Childs, Ashon Crawley, Josen Masangkay Diaz, Fatima El-Tayeb, Virginia Escalante, Rosiangela Escamilla, José Fusté, Jeff Gagnon, Joshua Guzman, Ren Heintz, Bernadine Hernández, Cheryl Higashida, Christine Hong, Grace Hong, Anita Huizar-Hernández, Meryem Kamil, Martin Kessler, Roshanak Kheshti, Jodi Kim, Ashvin Kini, Jim Lee, Chien-ting Lin,

Marissa K. López, Lisa Lowe, Maurice Rafael Magaña, Salar Mameni, Curtis Marez, Esteban Martínez, Melissa Martínez, Kelly Mayhew, Jim Miller, Natalia Molina, Alejandro Morales, Yumi Pak, Jade Power-Sotomayor, John Rieder, Joaquin Rios, Dylan Rodríguez, Cathy Ruiz, Rosaura Sánchez, Tom X. Sarmiento, Cathy Schlund-Vials, Davorn Sisavath, Amanda Solomon Amoral, Shelley Streeby, Thea Quiray Tagle, Josephine Talamantez, Meg Turner, Niall Twohig, David Vázquez, Kalindi Vora, Katie Walkiewicz, Robert Warrior, Tiffany Willoughby-Herard, Lisa Yoneyama, Lisa Yun, Salvador Zárate, and Diana Zuñiga. I wish to thank Chon Noriega, Rebecca Epstein, and Xaviera Flores at the Chicano Studies Research Center. I was lucky to have incredible interlocutors at the First Book Institute: codirectors Sean Goudie and Priscilla Wald, Ben Bascom, Jordan Carroll, Juliana Chow, Mary Kuhn, Katie Walkiewicz, Sunny Xiang, and Xine Yao. Bella Perreira's sharp eye on the entire manuscript was a gift; thank you for being such a fierce research assistant.

Many shared their time and knowledge at the level of archives and collections. I thank the staff at the Hawai'i State Archives, the Hawaiian Historical Society, and the archivists at University of Hawai'i Manoa, curator Elizabeth Schexnyder at the National Hansen's Disease Museum in Carville, Louisiana, and Dr. Selma Calmes, former chair of the Department of Anesthesiology at Olive View–UCLA Medical Center in Sylmar, California. Special thanks to Jason Weidemann, Zenyse Miller, and the production team at the University of Minnesota Press. I wish to thank the *Journal of Transnational American Studies* for publishing an early version of part of chapter 1, and Duke University Press for permission to reprint an earlier version of chapter 3, which was first published in *Captivating Technology: Race, Carceral Technoscience, and Liberatory Imagination in Everyday Life*, edited by Ruha Benjamin. For support to complete research for this book, I thank the Ford Foundation, the American Philosophical Society, the Center for American Literary Studies at Pennsylvania State University, the University of California Humanities Research Institute, University of Kansas, and UC San Diego.

Finally, I end where I began by thanking my families—chosen and not—for providing such models for being with each other, even when we are far apart. Mom and Dad (and Mia), you are always there when I need you. Hector and Eddie, I could not have wished for better companions to grow up and get into all kinds of trouble with. The Dons, the Kims, the Perreiras—thank you for mapping out new paths to walk. And to Bella, Dominic, and Joo Ok (and Noodle), you make my life a joy.

Archiving Medical Consent

How could I deflect the audience's gaze away from my own
body and toward their own, toward a history we all share?
—KEN GONZALES-DAY, *LYNCHING IN THE WEST, 1850–1935*

In spring 2018, the Smithsonian National Portrait Gallery and the
National Museum of African American History and Culture in
Washington, D.C., hosted an exhibit, titled *UnSeen: Our Past in a New
Light*. In press releases, the museum and gallery announced that
the exhibition "[brought] to the forefront African Americans, Native
Americans and Latino Americans to amend America's historical narrative."[1] Pieces in it represented how an optics produces what might be
described as a self-reflexive meditation on state institutions broadly—
with particular emphasis on museums and national archives. Several
art pieces on display reflected on the ways visual politics of U.S. national
histories directly and indirectly memorialize stories of freedom and liberty. In this framing, the vast yet illegible trace of records and documentation of racialized violence, coercion, and dispossession make up
what some describe as the archives of racial liberalism.[2] Exhibit pieces
reexamined those enduring structural events not as anomalous but
rather as the conditions of possibility, the materials and fabric that define the United States as an unfolding colonial and racial project. The
question the curators and artists sought to answer: Who is legible in,
and perhaps as, U.S. national memory?[3]

The *UnSeen* exhibit had been in development several years before
the election of Donald Trump in 2016. When it launched in 2018, however, the scene could not have been timelier. The national mall was full
of people protesting, seeking to name specific crises and demanding
change across the United States and beyond. Demands included abol-
ishing Immigration and Customs Enforcement (ICE), shutting down
all immigration detention centers, and direct challenges to climate

change denial.[4] It was difficult to enter spaces like the National Portrait Gallery without the context of political protest and perhaps without asking what, in 2018, it could mean to "amend" historical narratives at the level of national projects. How might national galleries, museums, or archives reorganize themselves differently?[5] They were undergoing profound transformations, but what work is done in centering absented bodies ("the unseen") as sites of new memory ("our past in a new light")?

Artwork in it, in other words, marked a cultural engagement with this historical moment as an unsettling of those narratives of violence and origin stories of the United States. The two featured artists of the exhibit brought these conversations into a sharp focus: New Haven–based painter Titus Kaphar and Los Angeles–based photographer and artist Ken Gonzales-Day. Kaphar's portraits focused on spectacular and hypervisible figures like Thomas Jefferson and Andrew Jackson by juxtaposing them with the mundane images of colonial and racial violence, often rife with missing faces and bodies carved out of the canvas. Gonzales-Day's images featured routine scientific work, images of medical instruments, representations of collecting human data and bodies, and facial molds. Gonzales-Day in fact notes in interviews that he spent years sifting through basements and boxes of national archives and museums, looking through, and looking for, artifacts and documents and origin stories of the United States.[6] He describes his work as a reckoning. Narratives of national history, through his art, are rewritten back into the historical record as the raw materials of, and the witness to, state-sanctioned violence.

Gonzales-Day's well-known exhibition *Erased Lynching*, from which the *UnSeen* exhibit drew extensively, portrayed photos of spectators at extralegal murders, where violated Latinx, Asian, Indigenous, and Black bodies had been violently killed in mob executions. Many of those original photos circulated through the U.S. Postal Service as postcards signed with notes to family and friends, but in these scenes the images are digitally reconfigured to bring not the violated body to the forefront (as the exhibit's title *UnSeen* suggests) but instead the gleeful expressions of white spectators posing for the camera.[7] With pieces such as *The Wonder Gaze (Lynching of Thomas Thurmond & John Holmes, Saint James Park, 1933, San Jose, CA)* (Figure 1), viewers are not confronted with the intended spectacle of white supremacist violence—the violated body—but instead they encounter the witnesses of that violence.

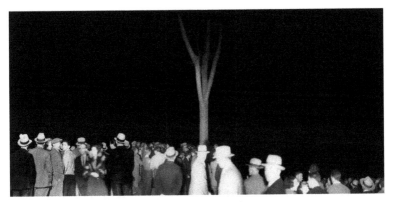

FIGURE 1. *Ken Gonzales-Day,* The Wonder Gaze (Lynching of Thomas
Thurmond & John Holmes, Saint James Park, 1933, San Jose, CA), *2006–17,*
Erased Lynching *series. Gonzales-Day's artwork removes the body from
the scene of a lynching at night. The tree and the crowd of white men and
women socializing while someone takes a photograph remain. Copyright Ken
Gonzales-Day 2006. Courtesy of the artist and Luis De Jesus Los Angeles.*

Wall-size photographs of mobs rearrange the scenes so that any museum viewer encountering those artifacts must study the faces in them,
compelling a kind of anthropological examination to explain the gath-
ering. A search for their own racial grammars, perhaps. Viewers face
the crowd, in a literal sense, and watch the watchers, study their looking.[8] For some, these rearranged photos draw attention not only to the
lynch mob but also to the significance of the surrounding landscape.
The tree at the center of the photograph serves as an anchor and disruptive perspective because it dominates over the crowd.[9] The images hail
viewers and call attention to the mundane backdrop of violence these
sanctioned acts allow. In the space of the National Portrait Gallery, this
featured exhibit names the unseen as an unspeakable violence, a central part of maintaining racial hierarchies under racial capitalism.

   Nicole M. Guidotti-Hernández's examination of lynching at the
U.S.–Mexico borderlands situates unspeakable violence as "fragments
of the very things selective memory bans from individual and national
consciousness."[10] While white racial and gendered violence produces
the conditions for long narratives of justice, as the layered and nuanced
historical conditions for social transformation, Guidotti-Hernández
argues that part of the work of interrogating racial violence and white

supremacy is in wrestling with an impulse to reproduce it in the form of resistance narratives. The representational problem regarding that form of violence is easily a reproductive (and reproducing) one, and yet traces remain detectable: "Clearly there but not allowed to be heard, seen, or experienced."[11] The formation of identities around such violence, she argues, can produce assemblages of meaning that resist reducing experience to binaries, making it particularly difficult to narrate those complexities through language or even visual culture. As she puts it: "When violence leaves its ineffaceable mark, it does not create merely a self-other relationship between violator and violated: rather everyone involved, spectators, enactors of violence, and the recipients of violence, is differentiated through [their] role in these processes."[12] The collective residues that make up abjection leave their traces, visible and invisible, unresolved.

Similarly, Koritha Mitchell argues that, because violence represented in lynching photos lays a particular authoritative claim to "truth" and evidence, turning to other forms—such as plays written by communities surviving extralegal racialized violence—provides other entry points into the past.[13] Gonzales-Day's other installations, for example, gesture to this representational problem by using photographs of sculptures, portrait busts, and ethnographic casts of Black, Indigenous, and Euro-American figures in museums, juxtaposing an anthropological impulse to measure nonwhite people, colonialism, and slavery through marble statues and likenesses. These images interrogate the role of scientific and medical studies, artistic modes of possessive remembering, the politics of ethnographic data, and a vast desire driving colonial and racial cataloging and world-building. Titus Kaphar, whose featured art was put in dialogue with Gonzales-Day's, took up the explicit contradiction of founding national narratives as the unseen in his 2014 dual portrait of Thomas Jefferson and a woman with dark brown skin, titled *Behind the Myth of Benevolence*.[14] The image of Jefferson, based in part on Rembrandt Peale's 1800 portrait of Jefferson, has been pulled back like a curtain—a canvas within a canvas—to expose a Sally Hemings representation peeking at the viewer from behind the canonical presidential painting. The original portrait of Thomas Jefferson is part of the White House Historical Association collection and suggests that this intertextual installation invited a layered critical engagement for anyone encountering it.[15]

Each artist interrogated public memorialization and the constructions of historical meaning in spaces like the National Portrait Gallery, marking its fiftieth anniversary with the *UnSeen* exhibit. It connected how those legacies are manifest in the present by gesturing indirectly to the Trump administration and Trump-era white nationalist resurgences, particularly as brazen and sanctioned expressions of xenophobia.[16] These conversations resonated within the discursive field of the exhibit as the terrain of racist violence over centuries, while at the same time symbolizing the unseen facts of history. The exhibit ultimately asked viewers to register the visual fields of white supremacy and racial hierarchy as they are reinforced through grammars of violence enacted on racialized bodies.[17] How those legacies structure the present, and how the National Portrait Gallery (NPG) stands as a representational problem and transmitter of national memory and knowledge production, was a driving force of the exhibit. On display was a reexamination of how racial orders are remembered and forgotten through sanctioned forms of state and extrajuridical violence.[18]

I open with this reading of the NPG because it embodies the contradictions of visibility in framing notions like personhood, consent, and representation, even as it obscures the central concern of this book: racialized forms of medical violence. The exhibit's critical engagements with scientific progress, however, elide the medical parameters undergirding constructions of humanity—its origin stories, parameters, and narrative possibilities—in the very framing of the "unseen."[19] *Archiving Medical Violence* reads U.S. racial formations through medicine and public health, and criminalized bodies and diseases, to present a critical engagement with cultural production, visual and literary texts, and imaginative texts taking up medicine and science. Doing so as contested sites, working within and against official narratives of racial capitalism, highlights the trajectory of public health from the nineteenth century into the mid-twentieth century as foundational to configurations of U.S. settler colonialism. Racialized violence in medicine and public health, in other words, emerges from this matrix. What constitutes violence in the context of the nineteenth-century colonized world shifts with the institutionalization of public health in the twentieth century, as the United States gradually adopts state antiracist frameworks and shifts in post–civil-rights discourse. Scholars argue that official and state-recognized antiracisms have worked to normalize deployments of power, attributing their usefulness to the transforming and differential relations of human value. Variations of human value, produced through racialized citizenship and personhood, mediate colonial and racial structures to recast through the lens of antiracism after the mid-twentieth century. The appearance of normative systems simultaneously allows for the naturalization of those categorical formations to be read as state management and not as part of an ongoing use of race to maintain differential power relations, what Jodi Melamed describes as "merely sort[ing] human beings into categories of difference."[20]

The representational problem of national memory and culture directly shapes how I attempt to reread the archives. Cultural and literary engagements with archives provide a critical lens through which to examine them—as a generative site of discursive power relations in public health and medicine, sometimes unsettling and sometimes shoring up those dynamics.[21] As medical archives present fraught and complex dynamics of racialization, attending to the ways literature and visual cultural production restage the archive points to the ways medicine and science are constitutive of settler colonialism, racial capitalism, and cultural politics. To place those conversations about cultural production within the field imaginary of ethnic studies also critically reengages the meaning of medical violence, therefore offering a critique of violence within medical imaginaries as a mechanism producing and investing in the discursive relationalities of race and criminality. Literature and cultural production are also generative for analyzing the ways the archives register and disseminate those discourses differently, critiquing the representations in cultural production as the very logics that produce and maintain them.

I am most interested here in mapping where these creative expressions unsettle official logics that produce meaning around progress narratives. Reading across sites of colonialisms, empires, and nation-states, several ongoing problems illustrate how narratives of race, memory, and violence have been operative as the raw materials of medical progress. I situate the project with several guiding questions. How has medicine conceived of, imagined, and incorporated criminality, incarceration, and the figure of the devalued, criminalized body into its frameworks—where incarcerated people, interned patients, and racialized quarantine communities are defined as coerced people across time and space who have been useful to advance medical science? In turn, how has this relationship shaped a broader understanding of race, colonialism, and their emergent notions of public health and public security? The book foregrounds the intersections of social identities in narratives of medical empire and nation-building, investigating not only the conditions under which prisoner-patients were used but also how they function as valuable figures when represented in the archive, in political life, in cultural production, and in collective memory. Across nineteenth- and twentieth-century contexts, I examine how tensions among categories and markers discussed in medicine—race, Indigeneity, criminality, and more—have also transformed across transnational and colonial contexts. I interpret the ways in which the figure of racialized prisoners and patients, devalued through criminality and race, has been revalued in medical and public health contexts.

Scholars of critical race and ethnic studies redefine medical histories as centering social and cultural politics to challenge enduring narratives of scientific progress, nation-building, and modernity, though deeper cultural analysis is needed to understand how criminality operates within this structure.[22] Those discussions document and often unsettle where medical and legal discourse intersect, unhinging easy notions of benevolence and scientific objectivity. Criminality, understood as a constitutive force for producing those haunting figures in archival and cultural artifacts, has not been thoroughly examined in the context of medicine and public health. One goal of this book is its relational starting point, studying racialization within medical and carceral contexts across nineteenth- and twentieth-century cases through medical research and writing. Beginning with the case of an incarcerated Hawaiian (Kanaka Maoli) in the 1880s, who was tried for murder and sentenced to death in the colonial courts of Hawaiʻi, the first chapter connects how this unfolds around the question of consent to be used as a human subject in deadly scientific experiments. In this chapter, the idea of consent presents a contested space in which to reconsider the politics of settler colonialism and sovereignty, particularly in the significant moment leading up to the U.S. government's illegal overthrow of the Hawaiian monarchy in 1893. Focusing on the imagined narratives and thoughts of the lead scientist researching the transmission of Hansen's disease (known historically as leprosy), and his ability to use an Indigenous prisoner-patient as raw materials in inoculation experiments, reveals particular logics of medicine that shape its racial trajectories long after the event.

The Carville Leprosarium in Louisiana, a case discussed in the second chapter, provides the spatial and temporal landscape for other narratives to emerge. Built on Houma ancestral lands and a ruined sugar plantation owned by Virginian Robert Camp, the United States National Leprosarium, for much of the twentieth century, found power as a triumphal institution in public health. Carville was formed out of national debates over whether Hawai'i ought to be understood as the nation's new scientific laboratory, as Congress redirected funding to support public health while local communities fought over having contagious communities nearby.[23] These discourses further find traction along the U.S.–Mexico borderlands in the early and mid-twentieth century, when Mexican and Mexican American communities in California were being criminalized through an emerging eugenics public health institution. Public health leverages the imperative to contain the spread of tuberculosis and other contagions across the United States, just as it continues to do so by securitizing and militarizing national borders.[24] Many scholars trace how the U.S. Public Health Service sought out its raw materials in these locations in its early formation and institutionalization, as well as in Tuskegee and in Guatemala City. As state-sanctioned acts, public and secret, what does reading across these structures, events, and their archives—holding them together and in tension—reveal about how public health is narrated, converging with race, settler colonialism, empire, criminality, nation-building, and public security?

This study also considers the figure of the prisoner-patient as an analytical focal point of comparative racialization. In archives, the figure of the prisoner-patient is consistently made and unmade as a prisoner and then refashioned as the condition of possibility for science and medicine—what a microbiologist in Hawai'i in the 1880s (and scientists and physicians for years after) thought of as the "human soil" necessary to advance modern medicine. Therefore, another goal of this study seeks to situate criminality and public health in the nineteenth century under such structuring contexts for carceral systems of the United States, as well as larger narratives that criminalize and devalue life. By drawing connections to extended networks of medical dialogue as they produce figures of colonial and racialized criminality, the chapters that follow attempt to move in and out of fixed categories of devalued life and civil death. Disease, contagion, and containment are also key concepts through which to interrogate the production of citizenship and social categories as a historically racial project. The central themes of *Archiving Medical Violence* focus on these social and political categories, from colonial contexts to emerging public health institutions of the twentieth century.

A third component focuses on cultural production and memory. An examination of literary and visual representation, as modes of critical memory and counterhistory, presents archival materials as cultural texts—all of which can be misread and redirected in ways that help make visible the manifold cultural politics at play.[25] Reading archives unconventionally means looking for how they speak and structure temporally unfixed modes of media and discourse. Locating in medical and scientific writing the speculative and cultural work done to articulate, undo, and revalue their own subjects in turn places diverse discussions, texts, and archives into an unexpected dialogue. This locates conceptual frameworks in biopolitical and necropolitical analysis, work emerging from the intersections of Indigenous, race, ethnic, and gender studies, prison studies, science and technology studies, and cultural theory. In reading the official scientific record, I interrogate not only a dominant perception of the role of medicine—that it is ultimately a benevolent and humanitarian project—but also the outcomes of archival knowledge. That is, the definitions of progress that are in play in scientific writings and their imaginaries and fields of vision become the materials of other possible futures. Reconsidering archival knowledge in this way—what it is, who it belongs to, and where it is sanctioned—sheds light on constructions anchored in racialist, ableist, gendered, and settler-colonialist logics that work to maintain those forms of knowledge production. In this context, I look to cultural production as that which reconfigures narratives of progress and individual freedom to consider what resistance and justice in the archive can mean, and for whom, and to do so without resolving the many contradictions that make it up.[26] The terrains of national culture are also sites of immersion into what Lisa Lowe describes as a repertoire of memories, events, and narratives, simultaneously locating spaces where hierarchical dynamics of social, legal, and political representation in the United States are worked out. *Archiving Medical Violence* points to those sites of collective memory to negotiate otherwise, taking for granted that culture has the

potential to rewrite those scripts—to shape how people forget and remember, to center expansive forms of resistance around refusal across
antiracist, feminist, queer, and migrant socialities.[27]

If culture provides a contested space to examine how narratives
structure such terrains—in the writing of histories, as well as other
authoritative discourses informing public health and security policies,
a logic that elides medical violence or reimagines it as progress for a
greater good—it might also be reconsidered as one in which "politics,
culture, and the economic form an inseparable dynamic."[28] The scope
of the book spans the late nineteenth century into the twentieth century because that inseparable dynamic is formed over time and against
what came before, what was residual and emergent, analyzing legal and
medical archives as well as cultural texts responding to them, to critically examine what I am calling *medical violence*. The notion of medical violence developed here conceptualizes a framework that presumes
legitimate or state-sanctioned forms of medical violence as an imperative for scientific and national progress. As the dominant narratives of
medicine also operate as benevolent, this book emphasizes violence
to resist the hypervisible categorization of individualized instances of
abusive, anomalous, or misguided medicine—the sadocriminal acts
carried out by rogue doctors and scientists discussed above.[29] Those
narratives have been incorporated into histories of violence. This book
instead foregrounds the intimate, mundane, and often invisible as another central story of violence. After 1884 in Hawai'i, for example, a man
sentenced to death was transferred to a doctor as a subject for medical
experimentation. Through this process, he became a focal point for articulating arguments that rationalized racial hierarchies for scientific
progress. This public, yet highly specialized, conversation about the
case unfolded in contemporary medical journals and popular magazines, such as the *British Medical Journal* and *Cosmopolitan,* from the
nineteenth century on. It also circulated as an ongoing conversation in
fiction, popular histories, and law. What the first chapter charts is how
this evolving narrative and its deployment in framing the U.S. nation-
state functions, over time, as a social and cultural question.

Archiving Medical Violence highlights medical violence through
the tensions of cultural production and memory, looking for productive moments of discord produced by the archive itself. Refashioned
around archives and literary forms, displaced by geographic locations,

and unsettled by temporal shifts that anchor memory, each chapter reads across official documents, novels, memoirs, and scientific writing to think anew social and political life surrounding the figure of the prisoner-patient—to interrogate the impulse to "study life as an object," as Kalindi Vora argues, as it emerges from medical violence.[30] The expansive collection of artifacts—such as cases and narratives that criminalize, devalue, and revalue life through medicine and a carceral state—provides a lens for reading its raw materials in colonized and racialized bodies. Medical history, at its center, is a sustained and uninterrupted presence of violence, and this book takes that narrative for granted to examine how culture reimagines and interrogates what that violence means as a relation of power. Focusing on the visual politics of race and medicine, I further demonstrate why race narrative matters in recasting antiracism through medicine, and what this means for how we imagine medical violence more broadly. Put another way, this Introduction maps a continuum for the chapters to work through at small and large scales, understood through the contested representation of bodies, locations, and recourses. Human bodies are examined as structurally similar, while not the same, to "land and natural resources . . . dispossessed in the period of capitalist growth during European territorial colonialism."[31] Beginning with the late nineteenth century, my approaches to archives and the problems emergent from historical sites, such as state archives and museums, foreground the centrality of those spaces for creating the official memory of medical violence.[32] Framing the archives this way raises questions about coloniality in relation to national memory, and in rereading as such makes visible a particular formation of race and the settler state in U.S. public health.

Unfit Archives and the National Remembering: The Case of Henrietta Lacks

As discussed above, the narrative framing of the *UnSeen: Our Past in a New Light* exhibition sought to "bring to the forefront African Americans, Native Americans and Latino Americans to amend America's historical narrative." What exactly does it mean, we might ask, to "amend" historical narratives at the level of national art projects? What work is done in centering absented bodies (the unseen) as a site of memory (our past in a new light) in those national institutions?[33]

What is the normative infrastructure of the institution's language and practices—and what contradictions emerge from state-sanctioned cultural events at the intersections of race, gender, sexuality, class, nation, and violence?[34] Read against other portraits in the museum—LL Cool J, Toni Morrison, and Michelle and Barack Obama—the gallery space laid claim to new possibilities for the public to imagine a different future in the nation's capital, which was reflected in how some news media narrated the event as a major shift in historical thinking about race, memory, and nation.

As if in search for answers to such unspoken questions the exhibit pieces were raising, NBC gravitated toward the 2017 portrait by artist Kadir Nelson, *Henrietta Lacks (HeLa): The Mother of Modern Medicine.*[35] Lacks was a working-class Black woman, tobacco farmer, and mother. After she was admitted to Johns Hopkins Hospital in 1951 as her health diminished and her cellular masses evolved into tumors, doctors removed and collected her cells without her consent or knowledge, tested them, and found them to be uniquely resilient. This led to scientists categorizing them as "immortal," signaling the immeasurable value they hold for untold future studies and unimaginable possibilities for humanity.[36] After her death in 1951, HeLa cells (a laboratory scientist's shorthand for Henrietta Lacks's cells) were cultivated and preserved, becoming the most widely used cellular material for medical research development. As many note, since Lacks's death, more HeLa cells exist in the world than ever existed in her living body.[37]

Nelson's rendition of Lacks, however, invites a different narrative. He depicts Lacks with a worn Bible pressed against her body and a wide-brim hat wrapping around her head. The backdrop of the portrait displays patterns spread across wallpaper resembling falling raindrops—or, perhaps, clusters of cellular material on a glass slide glowing through the light of a microscope. The colors and tones hint at a period prior to Lacks's death, before she was admitted to Johns Hopkins Hospital for the last time. The "maternal" figure of medical modernity gestures toward a forgotten memory, while also registering a legacy anchored in histories of race and nation, as much as it points to reproductive logics.[38] The portrait seems to also highlight other aspects beyond the now well-known narrative that produced the conditions of possibility for scientists to collect her cellular matter and discover their supposedly immortal characteristics—therefore proving its value to the futures of medical science. Looking to Henrietta Lacks this way, and how she is situated by the Smithsonian National Portrait Gallery through Nelson's portrait as "The Mother of Modern Medicine," suggests a reproduction and repurposed undercurrent of liberal multiculturalism as a distribution of antiracisms in the capital at a moment when Donald Trump's presence in the White House makes visible explicit and sanctioned racisms. A new form of an old racial order emerges, unfinished and ongoing, part of a centuries-old racial project. The portrait offers up a terrain of contested cultural representational landscapes.

The NBC News crew featured Nelson's piece and attempted to capture the "new energy inside these old walls," referring to critical engagements with race and the representation of Indigenous people and people of color in the gallery.[39] As the news anchor notes, this was a way to paint a "more complete picture" of U.S. history. When asked if the exhibit might be politically divisive, potentially presenting tensions for viewers that may be unwanted, a gallery spokesperson noted: "If it makes people uncomfortable that's okay. We want to be a space where critical dialogue can happen." As if to present evidence of the project's work of "fostering a new understanding beyond the art," the report shifts to patrons, filming a white woman and a Black man standing together and encountering each other for the first time. While they puzzled together at the image of Henrietta Lacks, the white woman put to words the contradictions the portrait seemed to elicit from viewers. She commented nervously on the dialogue it enabled with the person next to her: "We're new best friends! We enjoyed looking." Then, turning to the portrait of Lacks, she concludes: "My heart breaks for her. But look what she's done for the future." The statement echoes several moments in Rebecca Skloot's best-selling account of the Lacks family, *The Immortal Life of Henrietta Lacks,* most of which circle around Henrietta's daughter, Deborah Lacks.[40] In that narration, Deborah is represented as one of several family characters wrestling with how to put to words the value of their mother within and beyond a scientific futurity. Indeed, the book ends with an account of something like Deborah's last words: "But maybe I'll come back as some HeLa cells like my mother, that way we can do good together there in the world. . . . I think I'd like that."[41] Likewise, discussions about what justice means for the family moves from painful memories across generations, which include seeing the exploitation of Lacks for science when her family dealt with ongoing health, financial, and social pressures. Statements such as: "We ain't gonna get rich about any of this stuff on my mother cells. She out there helpin people in medicine and that's good, I just want the story to come out to where people know my mother, HeLa, was Henrietta Lacks," and "It's too late for Henrietta's children. . . . This story ain't about us anymore. It's about the new Lacks children."[42]

Certainly, Skloot's research, journalism, and publicity around her book provided the unseen story of Henrietta Lacks to come into view in ways previously impossible. At the NPG, while surrounded by hundreds of portraits and art pieces representing various moments of racial violence in U.S. history, the gallery's collections indeed appeared to reckon with epistemological shifts that attempt to name an understanding of U.S. history as a continuous colonial and racial project of violence. The details of Nelson's portrait in this case, however, prompted a response to incomprehensible narratives of medical progress. The explanation for racial violence in U.S. history finds power in medicine, not as a cause but as a lens for understanding what to do with that violence. In the process, other racist frameworks, such as the racial politics that undergird national origin stories, are short-circuited to make way for resolution, amendment, and the making sense of racialized violence through medical futures. On their own, Arlene Dávila suggests, representations do not challenge racism: "It takes structural change to create a visual revolution that can fully change and destroy our racist illusions."[43] What allows this sequence uttered by the white woman and captured by the news camera—"We're new best friends. We enjoyed looking," "My heart breaks for her. But look what she's done for the future"—is at once tethered to a condition of violence as progress and to the conditions of impossibility to see, by which I mean reckon with, other pieces representing forms of sanctioned violence hanging down the hall. They are hidden in plain sight.[44]

This book, then, is about the unseen as much as it is about the hypervisible. I began with a discussion of the Smithsonian and Nelson's portrait, and responses captured and archived in news media, because it encapsulates an encounter of medical-state violence as a cultural field perpetually mediating national memory and scientific futurity. Well-charted is the amplification, within the walls of an institutional space known to preserve and distribute an official national narrative, of the actuality that something was unfolding in the United States capital.[45] As Melamed suggests, racial cruelty, as both a material reality and an enduring concept of history, points to an "extreme or surplus violence alongside and within state practices of supposedly rational violence— military, security, and legal—through which the state establishes itself as at once the protector of freedom and an effective, because excessive, counterviolence to the violence of race."[46] What might it mean to reconcile or amend historical narratives of violence through the visual story of Lacks?[47] The language of inclusion perhaps instead reveals where race and medical science collide with national health as institutions of biopower.[48] In approaching the image of Lacks as a contradiction of history, at once folded into the incommensurable image of "The Mother of Modern Medicine," a location of materiality makes possible other nationalist speculations about its scientific narratives of history, memory, and futurity.[49] At a larger scale, when understanding U.S. history as violence—read through legal frames of amendments, corrections, humanitarianisms, or other progress narratives—the discussion that follows offers an alternative way of thinking about the racial grammars of the present.[50] The emphasis on how this story is told also invites looking through a particular lens to envision how techno-futures are imagined, as does the shifting relationships between science and the terrain of national culture.[51] In this sense, such a shift in focus points to how a structure of feeling in medical progress emerges in direct tension with—and is constitutive of—medical violence. The story of Henrietta Lacks—while over the past decade made a symbolic example of what mundane violence is and what it means for racialized, gendered medical subjects—points to other ways this conversation has shifted over time, signaling ongoing sites of struggle around what health produces for the state, how those meanings are created and maintained, and what groups are protected under those terms.

Archiving Medical Violence also considers how this kind of medical violence functions not so much as an anomaly in need of unique explanations but as continuously present in museums, in the storerooms of the state archive, as a representational politics in media, literature, on the big screen, and in television, and more broadly in the racial geographies of culture. The story of Lacks's violent encounters with medicine sits at these intersections, entwined in the political sphere of working out what subaltern stories can mean when on display in state and institutional spaces. This medical narrative signaled a hypervisible futurity in science laboratories and in speculative visions of capital as multimillion-dollar industries of biotech companies, as well as a usable pedagogical conversation in classrooms of medical and science students. The mundanity of this moment of sanctioned-violence-as-medical-progress, in other words, tells a different story that continues to hold sway over how bodies in the past are interpreted and interpellated into the present. This might be where reflection on emergent racial grammars, what Hortense J. Spillers describes as "the names by which [Black women are] called in the public place . . . signifying property *plus*," opens up other critiques of knowledge production.[52]

Consider again the white woman's comments about Lacks—"My heart breaks for her. But look what she's done for the future"—which were directed not at the image but at the person. As the curators and the artist have commented, the visibility of her life and her bodily contributions to medical science ought to register as an ethical and representational problem. That manifests in the museum by garnering attention and reflection on the racialized and gendered foundations on which medicine benefits "the public." Through centuries of extractive and predatory logics, this has been the condition of possibility for medicine to thrive and reproduce its own and others' futures. In other ways, though, it points to evolving conversations about the ways Lacks's story has been summoned into the present as part of a multicultural politics.[53] While attention to cultural production demonstrates the structuring of racist violence as illegitimate through multicultural liberalism, the incorporation of that violence finds new currencies in a neoliberal continuum. Interpreting the museum patron's statement through a critical reading of multiculturalism signifies a temporal tension in that Henrietta Lacks elicits something in the present rather than the past, activating continuous, ongoing significance felt now. The heart "aches," as a viewer suggests, compelled to feel what happened to Lacks but experienced by the viewer.[54] And what to make of the gesture to "our future"? What this book examines is how medical violence registers as rationalized progress by imagining the value of that violence forward and into the future.

Race and the Settler (Multicultural) State

A politics of representation in medicine under neoliberal multiculturalism raises other questions about why these discussions emerge differently than they have before now. How do definitions of privacy violations, refusal of consent, and ownership and property of bodily materials shift and transform over time and across race, gender, sexuality, and citizenship? Legal discourse provides ground upon which to uphold new forms of personhood, producing a figure by imagining, discussing, and anchoring bodies in narratives of race that stand for other iterations of power and state management. Neda Atanasoski and Kalindi Vora describe this process of disavowal as a type of stand-in, a techno-future signifying the human as the embedded relationality of racial grammars. The phenomenon manifests as surrogacy, they argue, foregrounding a spectrum of human substitutes that stretches across post-Enlightenment modernity. That surrogacy points to a continuum enfolding a multitude of activated figures across time and space: "the body of the enslaved standing in for the master, the vanishing of native bodies necessary for colonial expansion, . . . invisibilized labor including indenture, immigration, and outsourcing."[55] As a figure, the surrogate makes possible usable progress narratives, or a new history of biocapitalist life support.[56] Over a longer history across the globe, Atanasoski and Vora suggest that the surrogate also evacuates the violent conditions that produce them, recapitulating disappearance, erasure, and the structural forms of elimination "necessary to uphold the liberal subject as the agent of historical progress."[57]

Others framing this phenomenon through Indigenous science studies point to a contradiction of intersecting social and political realities. Kim TallBear argues that in unsettling colonial sciences through Indigenous sciences, the multicultural settler state as the overlooked site of ongoing colonial violence underpins a state project of "dreaming up" an ideal settler future in "inclusive and multicultural tones."[58] Medicine emerges (again) as settler-colonial projects making and measuring the parameters of the human in and against various publics (as public health, security, housing, goods, and resources). Furthermore, it does this while encoding colonial projects that identify those in need of protection and mark those in need of containment and management.[59] Interrogating such drives toward positivist narratives that anchor settler states, TallBear suggests reframing "dreams of progress toward a never-arriving future of tolerance and good that paradoxically requires ongoing genocidal and anti-Black violence, as well as toward many de-animated bodies."[60] Denise Ferreira da Silva argues that reorienting race as a global idea attends to other tensions. Developmentalist logics of scientific knowledge production situate race as the operative stand-in or surrogate for capitalizing on social fissures in the twentieth century, which are fundamental for maintaining and growing capital and profits. That global formulation of race presses on more static notions of racial formation in the United States, particularly those codified by law and historical developments of civil rights discourse.[61] Melamed locates this mode in the postwar reconfigurations of racial liberalism's imaginary of tolerance, and I build on these theoretical tensions to reconsider logics that produce the conditions for the commonsense hierarchical violence structuring life globally.[62]

To return to Kadir Nelson's portrait as one such cultural site working out the contemporary meaning of medical violence through multicultural logics, we might ask how this form of cultural production elicits the contradiction of surrogate humanity. To what degree does the portrait navigate developmental (i.e., historical, spatial, temporal) narratives of race? In the example of the white woman viewing the portrait, this affective response attempts to reconcile an aching heart through scientific futurity and technological progress. At the scale of one person in the National Portrait Gallery encountering the image, it can amend the American historical narrative through medical futurity. The imperative to "look at" what Lacks has done for the future as an implicit rationalizing of medical violence prompts the question: From the location of the nation's capital, who do we imagine mattering enough to have claim over this future? If this image interpolates Lacks as a surrogate for all humanity—a racialized and gendered mother of modern medicine— then to position her in relation to future publics, kinships, and contested definitions of justice within a racist settler state calls for other interpretive lenses to wrestle with this current moment. Imagined at the margins of the State's futurity, and otherwise not imagined with a future at all, the Lacks family in recent years has offered a kind of limit point to such forward-looking questions.[63] In 2018, Lacks's grandchildren challenged the nation's protection of biocapital and its claim on their ancestor's body when they brought a lawsuit to the U.S. courts to seek guardianship over HeLa cells. Their case raised the question as a legal problem for the courts to answer: "Can the cells sue for mistreatment, misappropriation, theft and for the profits earned without their consent?"[64] Under current U.S. laws, no one owns Lacks's cells because the patent process to transform them into property was not available to scientists at the time. Indeed, these mechanisms were supposedly not needed, yet understanding how they become the property of anyone who buys them points to an unspoken permission to sell, indicating some form of ownership in the first place. Such an act initiates possession and the right to sell without explicitly signifying a construction of property. The lawsuit sought to assert, in other words, a form of personhood as a challenge to the possessive logics of state medicine to claim racialized, gendered subjects as theirs to manage.

What makes this case unique for medicine, and a palpable concern about bioethics for a broader public, is that Lacks's body became immeasurably valuable for science under the backdrop of what might otherwise be understood as an individual moment of aberrant and misguided science in the Jim Crow South. The conditions for publicly naming the bioethical problem, that Lacks and her family were "misused," were material conditions: the unique cancer cells in her body that became known in the scientific world as HeLa cells.[65] The National Museum of African American History and Culture's website notes that Lacks "presents moral and philosophical questions around issues of consent, racial inequalities, the role of women, medical research and privacy laws."[66] The portrait of Lacks therefore provides "rich platforms for historical understanding and public dialogue," and its place and location suggest recognition of their weight and significance. At the same time, it functions as acknowledgment of a fraught and contested national memory that seeks to narrate the value of Black life. As part of a curatorial project, designed and administered by two major national institutions, the inclusion of *Henrietta Lacks (HeLa): The Mother of Modern Medicine* shifts attention to the question of who represents the nation in the symbolic space of the nation's capital. Lacks's story seemed to press on more complex symbols of progress and modernity around medicine, public health, and public protection. But what contradictions emerge when trying to reconcile raced and gendered violence with a desire for medical futures? This became such a contradiction while other conversations about how to reckon with U.S. history surfaced, such as the emerging reality of the Trump presidency and the firming up of white supremacist affect and xenophobic feeling in the United States and around the world.[67] Nelson's rendition of Lacks came into view during the aftermath of several moments of reorientation prompted by the election, while also marking embedded legacies of white supremacy that continue to make meaning of the United States in its most sanctioned, official spaces.[68]

In addition to privileged national sites such as the NPG, Lacks's story has engendered widespread consideration of the politics of her body elsewhere. Skloot's book, for example, became a teaching tool for a wide range of general students, from grade school to higher and graduate education. While I was studying at the University of California, San Diego (UCSD), *The Immortal Life of Henrietta Lacks* was adopted for general ed courses to have students wrestle with the bioethics of the case. UCSD is a university widely known for its research innovation in the fields of science and medicine, as well as its partnerships with the largest pharma companies, its privatized sectors of scientific and medical researchers, and its long connections to the military and war industry development. In 2011, Lacks's story in the mainstream prompted the Center for Ethics in Science and Technology in San Diego to initiate a colloquium entitled "The Henrietta Lacks Series," consisting of nine forums under the name "Exploring Ethics." These attempted to navigate the conversation with various publics around the best-selling book, led by experts in religious studies, biology, and the biotech industry. UCSD's Theater Department initiated a performance of Lacks's life, *Being Henrietta,* written by artist-in-residence Monique Gaffney, which dramatized her life, as well as marking the significance of it beyond the scientific value of HeLa cells, in relation to the ongoing discussion on campus.[69] Like Nelson's portrait, the story presented people and communities with an encounter with a medical crisis, offering entry points for thinking about the undercurrents that structure racial inequalities of the historical past unfolding in the present. Forms of racism that made race the organizing principle for Black life in the 1940s and 1950s continued to carry over into the world of medicine, logically and without much explanation. How is an enduring narrative of medical violence reconciled in scientific national memory? What investments undergird it as humanitarian and triumphal moments? The discussions were not new then, yet they brought Lacks and her family into the mainstream imaginary, with central notions of medical ethics and biomedical tension, raising a series of cultural problems to be worked out on a national stage in the capital of the United States. This plays out across the United States on university campuses, whose roles in scientific research make possible the reproduction of HeLa cells and the progress markers that give them value. Critics and journalists alike were quick to question how to understand the ethical choices made by those researchers who collected human materials, such as blood and tissue samples, from Lacks's family members without explaining why they were doing so.[70]

Furthermore, Alondra Nelson notes that Lacks's case ought to be understood in relation to U.S. global health and empire. In the same year that saw the publication of Skloot's best-selling book, the Obama administration was pressured to deal with the national and global implications of the uncovering of John Cutler's papers at the University of Pittsburgh, which documented extensive covert scientific syphilis experiments on imprisoned people in Guatemala. This major project was approved and funded by the United States Public Health Service and was carried out by renowned U.S. American scientists and doctors from 1946 to 1948. Cutler, in fact, was part of the Tuskegee syphilis experiments (discussed in the epilogue) and, throughout the twentieth century, found his way to various carceral sites with the most vulnerable groups made available to him in the name of scientific research. In recent decades, Black feminist science studies scholarship by Harriet A. Washington, Dorothy Roberts, Alondra Nelson, Ruha Benjamin, and others has set the stage for the story of Henrietta Lacks to be understood differently, not only read alongside major health policy reforms in the twenty-first century, such as the Patient Protection and Affordable Care Act, but also read historically and globally as a racialized and gendered cultural politics—drawing lines from the present to the Guatemala syphilis experiments, from Tuskegee to state health services for tribal nations, from plantations and prisons as research laboratories to surveillance and sanitation at the U.S.–Mexico borders.[71] These legacies continue to resonate with and affect lives today. Indeed, Alondra Nelson points out that "racially discriminatory practices in medicine have included Jim Crow healthcare facilities; a formerly segregated medical profession; stubborn health disparities evidenced by many indices; and 'unequal treatment' for blacks under medical treatment protocols for such conditions as cancer and heart disease."[72] The installation of Kadir Nelson's portrait of Lacks continues to spin out this narrative, and it does so as a national memorial seeking resolution and, we might read it, a resolution anchored in this contradiction: museum subjects are made visible in ways they could not be as medical subjects.

Chapters

That medicine structures fraught notions of consent, publics, health, and progress—directional forces that cannot be animated without supposedly willing subjects situated somewhere outside the category of "human"—is the central locus of this study. In the following chapters, I argue that public health and public security not only borrow from each other in constructing their own official narratives, but they also inform the production of racialized discourses that give meaning to the figure of the prisoner-patient. The silo of medical knowledge production also creates the conditions for cultural critique and interrogation through resistance, memory, and imaginative futures. Medical imaginaries and the social and cultural interrogations of medical science are coconstitutive, tethered and working in tandem with one another. What happens when, in Ferreira da Silva's words, these notions are deployed separately, and what happens when they move in conjunction? "There are only so many ways to account for the failed emancipatory projects that use race, nation, and culture precisely because we are not quite certain what happens when these notions are deployed separately or in conjunction with one another."[73] In this Introduction, I have tried to show that *Archiving Medical Violence* identifies an important site from which to understand how progress narratives are born of a modern project of racial liberalism—even though those narratives are not legible as such. The goal of the following chapters is to pursue that tension by charting the emergence and maintenance of such figures, as discussed above, across sites of coloniality and sites that demarcate nation-states and borders. Looking at such figures sheds a different light on too-often-overlooked or unseen archives of medical violence, on their formations at various geographical spaces, and the connective tissue in between. A map of the prisoner-patient is multisited and in transit, and it therefore presents a lens for understanding the transfer of medical knowledge across space, time, and scale. I follow scholars working in critical race and ethnic studies and transnational Indigenous studies who are interrogating logics of scientific settler colonialism and racial capitalism, placing the global fact of this movement as holding in tension the contradictions of space, place, temporality, and scale around how racial knowledge circulates, moves, and refashions.

As an entry point into questioning the archive, I also analyze the kinds of questions that evade inquiry in relation to the archive. I thus pursue the archive with three notions of recovery in mind: re-covering (covering over, overlaying, and obscuring) colonial power relations, re-covering (returning to view) to recenter social narratives that work to unsettle racial capitalism, and recovering (restorative), understood as a spatial-temporal insistence on healing, repair, and reparation. Lowe points to the ways archives and recovery premise how those are understood: "The process through which the forgetting of violent encounter is naturalized, both by the archive, and in the subsequent narrative histories," directs the kinds of questions that one can ask about those histories.[74] The archive is shaped and shaded by the emergence of liberal thought by way of global collisions of people displaced, enslaved, incarcerated, and devalued within the spectrum of social, cultural, economic, and political life. In turn, artifacts held in museums and state and national archives, such as many of those discussed throughout the following chapters, focus theoretical inquiry on notions of recovery. They question under what conditions notions such as freedom and unfreedom can be examined, how they put into play different valences of what recovery means and does, as Lowe argues. What does an intentional questioning of recovery register as "retrieval of archival evidence and the restoration of historical presence" and "the ontological and political sense of reparation"?[75] This notion works throughout each chapter as a politics of absence and presence in representational history. Interrogating concepts such as redress and justice not as given but rather as ontological, political questions elaborates possibilities of recuperation or the "repossession of a full humanity and freedom, after its ultimate theft or obliteration," troubling the notion of recovery as one anchored to forms of positivist historical analysis.[76] Full humanity is what is interpreted within rubrics of power, producing those conditions to interpret it as such, and it can be understood as insisting on reading the archive and its conditions of impossibility against itself. Lowe points to this paradox as what underscores "recovery as a question, and not as an established project or tradition." What remains lost in the question of a medical archive like this is the unmentioned notions of the term *recovery* as something that produces meaning under the lens of health and illness.[77] This book puts a kind of political and intellectual pressure on this theoretical framework of recovery to include not only a reading practice for official histories but also a practice of imagining archives as sites of useful contradiction.

The first chapter maps an engagement with the terms of recovery via the collision narratives in an 1884 criminal case of a Hawaiian man incarcerated for murder and sentenced to death. Addressing the stakes of this narrative and its location in the Hawai'i State Archives, the chapter provides a reading of the case and court conviction, its coverage and circulation in newspapers and in medical journals, and how similar accounts moved globally in colonial medicine to shape and refashion what the futures of public health could become. What made this case known to the world was, of course, not the crime of murder but rather how that provided the ground for social debts to be paid through medical experimentation. Microbiologist Edward Arning left Europe to work in Hawai'i under the Hawaiian Board of Health to study the transmission of Hansen's disease (leprosy). After reading newspaper coverage on the case, he requested to commute a death sentence to life in prison, arguing that debts to society could be paid by freely consenting and submitting to deadly inoculation experiments. Imagining a medical subject as the ideal "human soil" for scientific progress, doctors opened up a discursive field for narrating the necessity of acquiring medical knowledge through racialized criminality. Arning's report to King Kalākaua and the Board of Health sets the stage for what he, in at least one instance, calls "human soil"—and what I am calling medical violence. The medical scientists involved with the Board of Health were also political, economic, and social players working to dismantle Hawaiian sovereignty.[78] The implications of this experimental project continue to ripple across the globe and, as a result, captivate several watching publics. A coerced consent was given in exchange for a commuted sentence—the debt paid to regain life and a semblance of freedom—produced a usable vocabulary for medicine. The chapter centers the circulation of devalued life as a prisoner becomes revalued through medicine. It examines how those discussions were narrated as humanitarian—to advance science and move society from a premodern past to the modern present. The 1963 novel *Molokai*, written by microbiologist and medical historian O. A. Bushnell, unsettles the medical and criminal archive and asserts the first fictional account of the moment by accounting for several realms of the case as a structural event. This text reimagines, through a reading of the archive, the speech and thoughts of the characters of the moment, bringing to light several elisions and absences in the official record. *Molokai* is both an expansion of a settler-colonial archive—what David A. Chang describes as an enduring narrative of European discovery celebrating an "untroubled quest for knowledge"—as well as a questioning of methodological tensions in historical recovery, memory, and subalternity.[79] Reconsidering fictions against the figure erected in medicine offers a possibility for restaging the case—and more broadly the political and cultural implications of imperial medicine leading up to the U.S. overthrow of the Hawaiian monarchy. Together, the archive and the cultural engagement with it points to matrixes of conditions that produce devalued life, manufacturing a valuable human subject available for medical science.

The second chapter turns to the Carville Leprosarium in Louisiana to draw connections among colonial medicine, race, and the formations of a national public health institution. In the decade following the 1898 U.S. annexation of Hawai'i, debates in congressional hearings took place over how to carry out a long-term project to counter the spread of Hansen's disease and contagious diseases. Attempts to fund a leprosarium in Hawai'i failed despite territory designation through the Hawaiian Organic Act of 1900. Funding was eventually redirected to build the National Leprosarium in Louisiana. The U.S. Surgeon General Hugh S. Cumming, known for initiating the Tuskegee study of untreated syphilis in Black males in 1931, offered details on how the federal government acquired Carville and explained his reasons for engineering it as he did. The proposal worked through the pros and cons of designing the space modeled either after prisons (Angola Louisiana State Penitentiary would be one model) or something closer to a resort. Considering its origins before 1921, when the National Leprosarium was formalized as a national institution, the chapter places other narratives to situate it as a racial project. Not many years before that establishment, for example, existed the Indian Camp Plantation—a plantation of slave labor built on what the memorial narratives of Carville locate as Houma Indian lands. The first hospital was built in 1896 out of the unused slave quarters. Carville can be understood as a convergence of discourses working out entangled narratives of racialized criminality as a form of property and possession, and this chapter examines Public Health Service and congressional debates about race, as demonstrated by regular lines of questioning between Congress and U.S. Public Health officials, as the specter underpinning its production. The chapter examines memoirs, writing, and publishing at Carville, works and memories by patient-advocate Stanley Stein, former member of the Philippine Underground Resistance in Manila Josefina "Joey" Guerrero, and policy activist José Ramirez. The perspective these patients bring to the narrative of Carville navigates histories both official and from racialized, gendered subject positions.

The third chapter examines the role of prisoner-patient memory in recent Chicanx fiction. Reading Alejandro Morales's novel *The Captain of All These Men of Death* (2008) in tension with archives that document forced quarantine and experimental medical treatment at the Los Angeles Olive View Sanatorium and in Greater Los Angeles, the chapter shows how these narratives complicate our understanding of public health and safety as a nation-building project. In this way, it sheds light on the ways public health and public safety have converged both historically and culturally—a convergence that I describe as a carceral health imaginary. It analyzes the medical journal *California and Western Medicine*, along with interviews, news media, and cultural narratives representing patients' experiences in Morales's novel. By framing these texts, artifacts, and archives as contested and competing narratives, the chapter asserts that what is required in medical scholarship is a deeper engagement with culture and memory as sites of critical analysis and subalternity. It shows how such cultural texts, as counternarratives and cultural texts specifically interested in narrating as memory the experiences of Black and Latinx prisoner-patients, reimagine U.S. national history by linking global narratives of medical violence to ideologies of nation, progress, and national citizenship.

The epilogue expands the discussion on national memory and futurity begun in the Introduction. Specifically, it analyzes the significance of the 2010 uncovering of the U.S.-funded study of syphilis experiments on prisoners, soldiers, sex workers, and orphaned children in Guatemala. The long archival arc of the preceding chapters provides a platform for interpreting the uncovering of the syphilis experiments as an important entry point into what medical violence continues to mean for national memory of the United States in a global context. *"Ethically Impossible": STD Research in Guatemala from 1946 to 1948*, a 206-page interpretive report published in 2011, offers a way to consider how violence is currently being subsumed in the neoliberal multicultural moment and to connect the "value and valuelessness of bodies to the value and valuelessness of [medical] belief systems and social worlds."[80] In that text, the committee—composed of historians, medical experts, and legal scholars—presented to President Obama their nine-month "thorough fact-finding investigation" into the specifics of the U.S. Public Health Service–led studies in Guatemala, involving the intentional exposure and infection of vulnerable populations. The epilogue demonstrates the concerns of the book as a contested history of the present, situating the syphilis experiments against an imaginary of the nation-state that cannot reconcile its own histories of violence. Instead, what emerges is a clearer sense of how medicine has reconciled legacies of violence outside its borders, raising the question of the limits of U.S. standards when research travels across oceans or just across the border.

What this constellation of thought means for antiracism—how it is deployed in the current moment as well as into the future—depends on how it has produced meaning in the past and how critical memory and creative futures shape those pasts.[81] In the twenty-first century, new spaces for people of color and Indigenous people collide with, and are unsettled by, expressions of self-determination and by collective futurities.[82] Creative expression, including novels mediating the official archive to navigate a racial discourse of their moment, provides space for thinking through those decolonial tensions. And yet, the final stages of this study emerge from a moment that is creating new forms of racism, xenophobia, policing, extraction, environmental threats, and dispossession, as well as radical possibilities that continue to respond to those new forms. A post-Obama, Trump-era carceral health crisis—prompted by, many argue, a capitalist logic undone in the aftermath of the novel Coronavirus in 2019—sees new configurations forming around white nationalism, anti-Asian racism, devalued Black, Brown, and Indigenous life in prisons, at borders, in meatpacking factories, and in hospitals.

This highlights a continuum around an enduring death toll that charts ongoing forms of racism and white supremacy, manifest while many of us write, think, teach, and work.[83] It moves the moment far beyond a postrace story and into a future that has been structured by race, yet is always reimagined otherwise.

CHAPTER 1

Medical Violence, Archival Fictions

I have linked as similar ideas in the motives accompanying my application to His Majesty's Privy Council to be allowed to perform some inoculation-experiments on the condemned convict Keanu. The application I made resulted in the sentence of death passed on the murderer being commuted to penal servitude for life. With the prisoner's written permission I commenced operations on the last day of September 1884.

—DR. EDWARD ARNING, *REPORT OF EDWARD ARNING, M.D.,*
ON LEPROSY, NOVEMBER 14, 1885, SUBMITTED TO
KING KALĀKAUA AND THE HAWAIIAN BOARD OF HEALTH

Suppose for a moment, that Keanu had reasoned thus: "I readily submit to inoculation with leprosy, not only because I shall save myself from immediate death, but also for a higher reason. I have killed one man, and deep is my sorrow; should I by this inoculation become a leper, such a result may tend to save the lives of many."

—RECTOR H. P. WRIGHT, "THE INOCULABILITY OF LEPROSY,"
BRITISH MEDICAL JOURNAL, 1888

The medical archive structures the events encountered in it. And the categories falling under the term *medical* overlap with other forms in the archive, whether they are cataloged under court and criminal cases, property, deeds, and land titles, ancestries and genealogies, or maps and photos. These constitute the organizational parameters of its colonial structure. The formation of the archive might then be read as just that, a formation, and therefore reading, rereading, and misreading its form offers a way of grasping the elusive logics of racial liberalism.

In *The Intimacies of Four Continents,* Lisa Lowe provides several critical readings of colonial and state archives that, through the readings
themselves, present a hermeneutics specifically attuned to the contradictions that give meaning to the archive:

> In examining state archives out of which these historical narratives
> emerge, I observe the ways in which the archive that mediates the
> imperatives of the state subsumes colonial violence within narra-
> tives of modern reason and progress. To make legible the forcible
> encounters, removals, and entanglements omitted in liberal ac-
> counts of abolition, emancipation, and independence, I devise other
> ways of reading so that we might understand the processes through
> which the forgetting of violence encounter is naturalized, both by
> the archive, and in the subsequent narrative histories. In a sense, one
> aim of my project is to be more specific about what I would term the
> economy of affirmation and forgetting that structures and formal-
> izes the archives of liberalism, and liberal ways of understanding.
> This economy civilizes and develops freedoms for "man" in modern
> Europe and North America, while relegating others to geographical
> and temporal spaces that are constituted as backward, uncivilized,
> and unfree. Liberal forms of political economy, culture, government,
> and history propose a narrative of freedom overcoming enslave-
> ment that at once denies colonial slavery, erases the seizure of lands
> from native peoples, displaces migrations and connections across
> continents, and internalizes these processes in a national struggle
> of history and consciousness. The social inequalities of our time are
> a legacy of these processes through which "the human" is "freed" by
> liberal forms, while other subjects, practices, and geographies are
> placed at a distance from the "human."[1]

One such illuminating case occurred in the 1880s in medical journals, in which scientists and others debated the life of an incarcerated man, Keanu, and the "contagious nature of leprosy" devastating
the Kingdom of Hawai'i.[2] The Supreme Court of the Hawaiian Islands
charged Keanu with the killing of a farmer, "one Charlie, a Japanese, on
the February 16th, 1884 at Kohala, Hawaii."[3] On July 9, 1884, Chief Justice
Albert Francis Judd delivered a guilty verdict of first-degree murder.[4]
The convicted would be hanged "within the walls of the [Oahu] prison"

on October 28, 1884.[5] The *Pacific Commercial Advertiser* referred to the event as "The Kohala Murder Case" and described the murder as an unfortunate moment of meaningless violence: "There was no quarrel, no cause, except the bloodthirstiness of a beast of a man."[6] Keanu petitioned for his sentence to be commuted to life in prison, which was denied. Dr. Edward Arning, a German microbiologist who was brought to Honolulu by the Board of Health, submitted a special request to King Kalākaua's privy council to permit the use of his body for experimental leprosy inoculations. Arning promised to "really advance our knowledge of the obscure disease."[7] The privy council meeting minutes reflect the interest in the case: the "committee to whom was referred the petition of Keanu for a commuted sentence, presented their report recommending that the petition be granted, in view of the valuable results to be obtained by experiments upon him respecting the action of leprosy."[8] The request was approved. With written consent, a notion that I trouble later in the chapter, Keanu was transferred to Arning's ward to begin the experiments. The doctor removed a "leprous nodule" from the cheek of a nine-year-old girl to surgically insert the mass into Keanu's arm.[9] Keanu began feeling rheumatoid pains within a month and "the cubital nerves began to become obstructed, this lasting until the 5th to the 8th month."[10] On September 25, 1888, Keanu was diagnosed with leprosy and transferred from the Oahu jail to Kalaupapa, Moloka'i, the quarantine site created under the authority of the 1865 Act to Prevent the Spread of Leprosy.[11] He remained there until his death in 1892.

This chapter examines that case as an event of deep cultural significance produced in the archive, as well as multiple and ongoing subsequent historical and cultural narratives. Indeed, the figure of Keanu—as opposed to the historical person—takes on a life of its own in medical imaginaries, finding its way into the discourse of law and public health, as a precedent for other justified forms of medical violence, as well as imagining forms of humanitarianism. Many scholars, historians, storytellers, novelists, museums, and state archives have narrated the contentious meanings of leprosy (Hansen's disease) in Hawai'i, often navigating Arning's research as a backdrop to the structural violence occurring, primarily surrounding sustained attacks on Hawaiian sovereignty.[12] Historian Kerri Inglis describes leprosy as a disease set apart, above all others that have affected the islands,

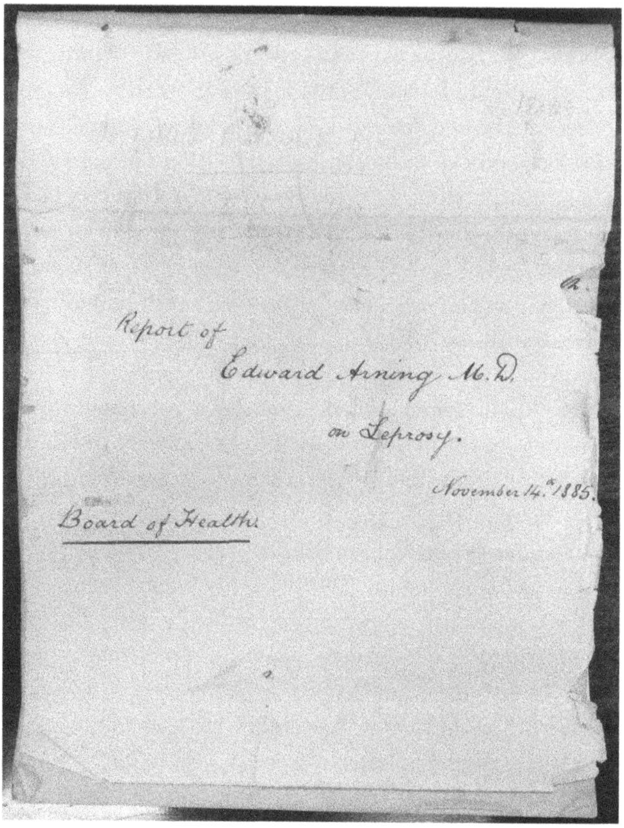

FIGURE 2. *Cover page of Edward Arning's assessment of Hansen's disease in 1885, which reads: "Report of Edward Arning M.D., on Leprosy. November 14th, 1885. Board of Health." Series 334–35, Folder "Dr. Edward Arning: 1883–1888," Board of Health, Hansen's Disease, Hawai'i State Archives.*

because it is a disease stigmatized for so long that it has been generally approached as "to be feared rather than to be treated."[13] Regardless of its exceptional history, however, criminalizing Hawaiians through leprosy should be understood within the context of the Hawaiian monarchy and people's resistance to colonial pressure, which included political and economic shifts since the early 1830s.[14] The Act to Prevent the Spread of Leprosy appropriated substantial funding and land seizures and authorized near limitless police power to the Board of Health "or its agents" to arrest "all leprous patients who shall be deemed capable of spreading the disease of Leprosy."[15] Neel Ahuja similarly examines medical writing, photography, and discourse surrounding leprosy that foregrounds the weaponizing of "the state's health policing power," as well as patients' activism to resist it.[16] The operative focal point for much of this scholarship has been about mapping the convergences of public health, disease, empire, and racialization—in particular as it undergirds colonial medicine and social life. While studies have examined the cultural circulation of Hansen's disease, emphasizing more the historical and legal artifacts of newspapers, acts, and U.S. violence, fewer studies have taken up the writings of medical scientists and fiction that emerge from this moment. And even fewer have discussed the cultural significance of the specific case of Keanu, the Native Hawaiian prisoner who was used in experimental inoculations in the 1880s—examined not only as a historical event that occurred publicly yet escapes histories of Hawai'i outside of the medical context, but also as a cultural flashpoint that shapes medical discourse about what can be imagined as fully human.

From Hawai'i to Trinidad, England, and back to Hawai'i, science writers in journals, magazines, and newspapers depict Keanu as an essential idea for medical professionals to navigate and negotiate definitions of race, coloniality, consent, criminality, and personhood. In some cases, the circumstances of Keanu prompted a medical impulse to imagine his thoughts and to rationalize the use of his body for fatally experimental procedures. Such a knowledge exchange represents an ongoing move to mediate sanctioned violence through the language of humanitarianism and benevolence, where, in the case discussed here, the notion of consent in which Arning and others anchored their claims to Keanu are tethered to the understanding that submitting one's own racialized, criminalized body to science constitutes an acceptable form of societal debt-settling. What it provides is the opportunity for medicine to advance knowledge globally, while the conditions that produce Keanu as a racialized criminal hinge on settler-colonial discourses structuring the scene—the very same that bring Arning to Hawai'i to research a cure for the disease.[17] Arning's initial motivations to travel to Hawai'i, it is important to note, were twofold. The primary reason was to research the contagious nature of leprosy, and the secondary reason was to collect photographic data on Native Hawaiians, a project funded by the Humboldt Institute of the Royal Prussian Academy of Sciences. The institute commissioned him to "make a study-tour to Hawaii for the joint purpose of investigating leprosy and acquiring an 'ethnographic collection.'"[18] In 1967, in one of the earliest critical examinations of Arning's research, medical historian and novelist O. A. Bushnell notes that if such a state-funded project were proposed in that moment it would have been greeted with "suspicion if not with horror in an application for a research grant today."[19] While the contemporary writing about Keanu's motivations for consenting to the experimental inoculations painted him as a guilty murderer who would do anything to avoid state execution, the event might also be read as a complex negotiation of colonial legal power relations. Being attentive to settler-colonial law, business, and medicine, which remade Keanu as criminal from multiple angles—as a murderer, as a patient infected with a criminalized disease, and as a colonial subject—at the same time opens the archive to be read against itself.[20] Reading the medical archive as an economy of consent raises several questions.

In the decade following the initial inoculations, Arning and Keanu became internationally known in journals and popular media, and this sensational narrative affected policy, public health regulations, and medical practices.[21] Popular magazines and medical journals, as well as journalistic and fictional representations, deploy—and occasionally unsettle—racialized, criminalized narratives of Keanu.[22] Soon after the initial experiments, news traveled to the Caribbean and caught the attention of Dr. Beaven Rake, the Trinidad Leper Asylum medical supervisor. On August 20, 1887, Rake published an article entitled "Leprosy and Vaccination" in the *British Medical Journal*. The journal provided the platform for physicians and scientists across the globe to weigh in on the Keanu case, as well as comment on their own and other medical experiments. When the details of Keanu's case reached Trinidad, Arning's work was already perceived as groundbreaking and as a valued precedent in colonial medicine.[23] Rake interpreted this value against unsuccessful scientific attempts to identify, through nonhuman experimentation, how *Mycobacterium leprae* was transmitted. Charting a global effort by imperial scientists documenting their research in journals, Rake wrote: "Seeing that inoculation experiments on various animals with leprous material (tubercles, pus, etc) in different parts of the world—Spain (Neisser), England (Thin), Hawaii (Arning), and Trinidad (*loc. cit*)—have hitherto failed to transmit leprosy, I think one is justified in arguing *a fortiori* that vaccination with pure lymph is incapable of doing so."[24] Rake discovered in the Keanu case the discursive space to mark a particular kind of medical value in colonized, racialized bodies. Rationalizing an institutional move away from failed animal experimentation, he championed prioritizing experimental work on human subjects—what Arning himself described as "human soil."[25] "I have had no hesitation," Rake declares, "in vaccinating both my own children out here [in Trinidad] from native arms, Hindu and negro."[26]

The case articulates legal, medical, and cultural notions for producing the discursive figure of what I am describing as the prisoner-patient—a figure emergent from conditions across several imperial medical conversations and practices in Hawai'i, the Caribbean, and England in the late nineteenth century. Keanu's consent to participate in these procedures—likely represented by an *X*-mark signature, such as the *X*-mark made on his criminal case court documents—provided the mechanism to commute his death sentence to life in prison and to discursively transform Keanu into another kind of subject: Arning's prisoner-patient.[27] Reading Keanu's consent not simply as an act of agency in relation to colonial medicine, as many did in medical and scientific communities in order to justify the experiments, but rather as an expression of contradictory colonial violence presents a different story than the one in the official record. Following the body of transnational scholarship that foregrounds the movement of not only people and bodies across borders and oceans but also ideas, cultural discourse, and knowledge production, this exchange unfolded as a global conversation, moving across empires through colonial medicine. Perhaps most notable in this discussion is the fact that it represents a multisited and temporally unfixed medical public where racial hierarchies are made visible within the historical conditions of colonialism, racial capitalism, and the maintenance and naturalization of whiteness as a possession.[28]

Accounts of Keanu's case in the *British Medical Journal* and other journals, newspapers, and books consistently describe him with the same biographical details. He was "a murderer in Hawaii, named Keanu," "the convict Keanu," the "Sandwich Island convict," "a condemned murderer," and, as one widely read history of Hansen's disease frames the case, "Keanu, the Murderer."[29] The documents reporting on Keanu located his "criminal" status or his Hawaiian identity (often

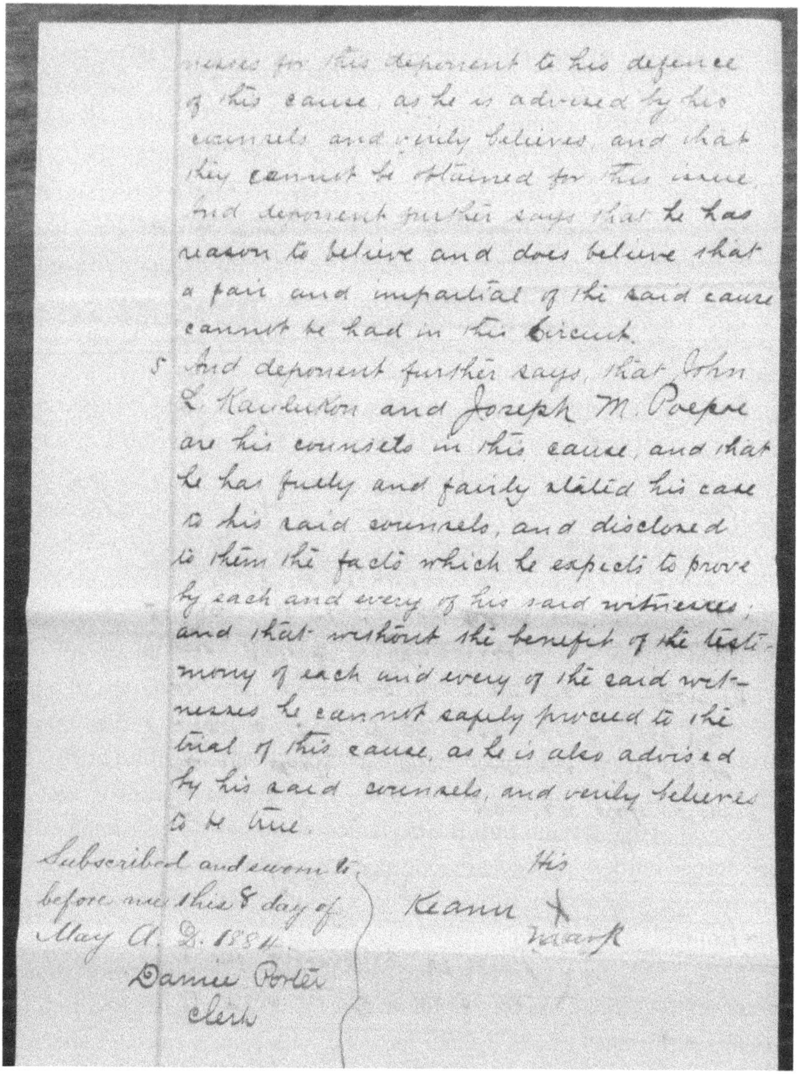
nesses for this deponent to his defence of this cause, as he is advised by his counsels and verily believes and that they cannot be obtained for this issue. And deponent further says that he has reason to believe and does believe that a fair and impartial of the said cause cannot be had in this Circuit.

5 And deponent further says, that John L. Kaulukou and Joseph M. Poepoe are his counsels in this cause, and that he has fully and fairly stated his case to his said counsels, and disclosed to them the facts which he expects to prove by each and every of his said witnesses; and that without the benefit of the testimony of each and every of the said witnesses he cannot safely proceed to the trial of this cause, as he is also advised by his said counsels, and verily believes to be true.

Subscribed and sworn to before me this 8 day of May A. D. 1884.
Daniel Porter
Clerk

His
Keanu X
mark

FIGURE 3. *A court order where Keanu was asked to provide his X-mark, May 8, 1884, which was signed next to the clerk Daniel Porter. "King vs. Keanu: Motion to Change Place of Trial," May 8, 1884, Box 1052: Criminal, Folder 002: Criminal Case Files of the First Circuit Court, Hawai'i State Archives.*

both) as central for justifying the medical procedures.[30] To return to Lowe's analysis above, this takes for granted economies of affirmation and forgetting and the ways they formalize archives of liberalism, therefore stabilizing a claim to civilize, to develop freedoms for some while "relegating others to geographical and temporal spaces that are constituted as backward, uncivilized, and unfree."[31] To read the archive produced around Keanu's case against itself is, in part, to reckon with settler-colonial logic guiding a medical community to situate racialized bodies as the raw materials for advancement.[32] The value of the body, especially when conflating the category of "human" with the category of "free," is linked to persistent narratives that spatially and temporally demarcate Indigeneity from conceptions of modernity.[33]

The constitutive processes informing the ideological formations of modernity in the context of Keanu's case provided a special moment for science and medicine. That is, racializing the figure of Keanu outside of modern time situates it against liberal accounts of the "human"; at the same time, it constructs life as criminal and, therefore, possessed by the state. As such, life is perceived as usable as a precariously situated body to benefit modern subjects. Aileen Moreton-Robinson, in formulating the emergence of white possessiveness as a narrative force within modernity that defines itself against Indigeneity, argues that possession over land, property, wealth, or one's very body, thoughts, and actions requires "a subject to internalize the idea that one has proprietary rights that are part of normative behavior, rules of interaction, and social engagement."[34] Moreton-Robinson's critical analysis of Western modalities of "the modern" helps to locate possessiveness as a discourse that makes possible the necessary revaluing of Keanu's racialized and criminalized body, but in particular when presented as existing outside the parameters that would otherwise define bodies as human.

As several of the medical reports on his case note, Keanu had been awaiting his execution date when asked to consent to these experiments. In an 1888 *British Medical Journal* article, for instance, entitled "The Inoculability of Leprosy," author H. P. Wright justifies Arning's decision to use Keanu this way. A rector of Greatham Parish in England, prolific author on colonial diseases, and champion of the British Empire, Wright upholds the sovereignty of the British state as the foremost authority to "grant" or "take [the] life" of a criminalized body for the sake of the "civilized nations."[35] In a statement that narrates biopolitical state imperatives, Wright calls on the state's sovereign power to justify medical violence against Keanu.[36] He insists on the state's moral right to kill: "The State, which could take life for the terror of evil doers, could also grant life in order to stay, if possible, in some degree, the advance of the most terrible disease that tortures man."[37] By Wright's account, which I examine in closer detail below, the constant threat of this "most terrible disease" provided the state the necessary grounds to narrate Keanu out of modern time, especially when such action protected and benefited a fully human white citizenry, emerging and solidifying as a "new subject into history within Europe."[38] By placing Keanu within this criminalized "prehumanity," Wright's justification serves to inscribe criminality and Indigeneity as prehuman existence. In Wright's shorthand, this is meant to signify the qualities of the "evil doer." While this situates Keanu as a racialized and criminalized subject existing outside of modernity, it also places him within a "modern" time just enough to hold him criminally culpable for crimes against society.

Perhaps this is how we can read this medical archive against itself. Colonial relations have been at the heart of European philosophical notions of human freedom, and rereading it can critically unsettle the "unevenly inhabited and inconsistently understood aftermath of these obscured conditions."[39] The archive absorbs colonial medical violence within those narratives of modern reason and progress, constructing differentiated humanness, (un)freedoms, and racialized criminality as a discursive space to great effect. The body maps value and utility, and it does so, following Jodi Byrd, across spatial and temporal transits of empire.[40] The figure of Keanu is made and remade, narrated and revalued for medical colonial science, particularly within the public platform of scientific writing. Conjuring such a figure is indicative of the conditions that produce the language of consent and the larger production of liberal humanism and autonomy. Scott Richard Lyons, examining the X-mark within a matrix of Native assent to treaties, describes this as "the agreement one makes when there seems to be little choice in the matter."[41] Those discourses helped produce the figure of Keanu as a liberal, autonomous subject—important for narrating a figure who possesses and is in control of his own body only enough to consent to giving it over as payment and for the advancement of medicine.

Tracing criminality, racialization, and settler colonialism restages

this event as a series of entanglements moving beyond the constructions of consent offered up at the time of Keanu's inoculations and
eventual death. In this framing, his body finds its early articulations
within legal and historical constitutions entwined with questions of
sovereignty.[42] Luana Ross connects criminality and sovereignty in her
work on criminalization in Montana, asserting that the production and
deployment of Native American criminality is intricately tied to not
singular but manifold discourses on sovereignty, noting the disruptive
impacts of formal and informal federal and state policies that "chipped
away at the sovereign status of Native people."[43] Through various state
and federal procedures, U.S. law consistently defined Native people as
"deviant" and "criminal" as a way to undermine rights to land through
racial criminalization and systematic incarceration.[44] Racialized bodies within this binary structure become legible as either citizen or criminal, as a part of or apart from the nation, and as subjects are divided
into naturalized categories of those who belong, those who need to be
contained, and those who can be used to maintain those categorical
divisions. In the late nineteenth century, the *British Medical Journal*
provided the discursive platform to work through and reconfigure
such notions of criminality and value, while also serving as a venue
for talking about human experimentation even as it naturalized those
discussions as acceptable, even humanitarian. Across the Pacific and
through colonial sites, it also made natural the practice of observing,
experimenting on, imagining the thoughts of, and literally speaking for
medical subjects.

Two essays published in one of the many medical journals on
Keanu produced in late nineteenth-century England illustrate this
process. H. P. Wright—English rector and prolific writer of lay medical
commentary—documented the public production of Keanu as a usable
subject for medical experimentation in his publications on preventing
Hansen's disease from infecting European nations. Wright's 1890 article
"The Inoculability of Leprosy" signals how those speculative accounts
of what Keanu might have thought when he consented to experiments
illustrate the production of a figure. This figure ultimately provides the
conditions of possibility for legitimized medical violence at that moment and even finds ground as a legal precedent in future justifications
of human experimentation.[45] I examine the contradictions between
articulating a racialized and criminalized figure as both imprisoned—

and, therefore, an available body under the care of the state—and at the same time free to consent to experimental inoculations.

Arning chose Keanu as, in his view, an ideal subject for medical experimentation because, among other factors, he was "a large, well-built Kanaka, to all appearances in robust health."[46] His descriptions of the ideal medical subject are telling. Arning notes that the experiments required not only an uncontaminated subject but also a place (land) that can be said to be largely untouched by disease, revealing the degree to which the doctor's own thinking was influenced by the ideas surrounding possession, the self, and property as it is constituted by empire. On the issue of contagion, he admitted in correspondence with H. P. Wright that the question "could only definitely be settled by the inoculation of a healthy individual of untainted nationality in a country free from leprosy."[47] Trained under German microbiologist Robert Koch, who was famous as the scientist who isolated the bacterial causal agents of cholera and tuberculosis, which ultimately won Koch the Nobel Prize in Physiology and Medicine in 1905, Arning adopted Koch's then-experimental methods for his own leprosy inoculations. Initially, this meant experimental trials with potato slices, gelatin, and eventually guinea pigs for his raw materials. When those materials did not work, he aggressively sought the human subject option—a medical subject he at one point describes this way: "As every seed requires its peculiar condition of soil, atmosphere, etc., to allow it to strike . . . so does the leprous germ . . . [need] human soil."[48]

Arning's descriptions of the ideal subject, announced without reservation, point to the regularized documentation of human experiments.[49] As a result, the concern over Keanu's physical and mental health, and status as a murderer and criminal, loomed large in the medical imaginary and regularly comes across as haphazard scientific speculation. Published images, charts, and written dialogues trace Keanu's family genealogy, guessing at whether Keanu might have had contact with Hansen's disease in earlier periods of his life; scientists researched and argued over his status as a "clean" subject for over a decade after the initial procedures—all in the effort to categorize Keanu as an untainted subject. Questions about the status of Keanu's family, including his son and nephew, became important parts of the contentious genealogical story that charts the transmission of Hansen's disease as either hereditary or as a contagion.

In the 1890 article "The Contagious Nature of Leprosy," for instance, sketches of Keanu, his son, and his nephew serve to map anxieties around kinship, heredity, and disease, accompanied with descriptions of their biometrics, general health, and how advanced their cases were. The author of the article points out that Keanu's death sentence "was commuted on condition that he submitted to the experiment [and much] interest was attached to the case, as it seemed to be one in which the appearance of the disease was only to be accounted for on the supposition that it had been communicated by the inoculation of leprous matter. It was stated that there was no history of leprosy in his family."[50] Photographs in Arning's personal ethnographic research in Hawai'i, which was created before and during his experimental work on Keanu, from 1883 to 1886, document people and places as exotic subjects, reproducing scenes in living spaces in the anthropological colonial gaze. The overlap between these efforts and the visual record in the medical archive, however, is also telling.[51] One photo in Arning's personal collection, entitled "Keanu, Hawaiian, frontal full figure," is of Keanu wearing only a steel shackle around his right wrist. Standing with arms tightly beside his hips, it suggests medical documentation for tracking various stages of Hansen's disease, yet the photo was kept as part of his ethnographic collection. The shackle further suggests that the image was taken immediately after Keanu was taken from the Honolulu jail, though no such notes or details are available. In contrast to such medical photographic images, taken, presumably as part of Arning's attempt to document the stages of the experiment, is a sketched image of Keanu produced two years after the initial experiments. The image depicts Keanu's fingers wrapped in bandages meant to protect the parts of the body that are numb, unfeeling, and exposed. But the dark patch on Keanu's arm, roughly one inch long and half an inch wide, is perhaps the most significant detail of the illustration, as it marks the original inoculation procedures.

Appearing in the second column opposite a description of Keanu, the sketch accompanies an essay that also details his age and physical state, the accounts of the accidents he suffered while detained in the hospital due to "attacks of vertigo," and his appetite and mental state.[52] Regarding his mental and physical condition, the author of this article comments: "The prisoner was then suffering from bruises of the face, head, back, and lower extremities, received by falling down a metallic winding staircase in the gaol at Honolulu during a fit."[53] The article continues by mapping a visual and biometric sketch, noting that his nephew was also a patient in the same hospital ward, with a bed next to Keanu's. The twenty-year-old son of Keanu's deceased sister is described as "a far advanced tubercular leper, covered with sores, almost blind, nearly deaf, and utterly helpless." Finally, the report identifies several family members with illnesses, as well as Hansen's disease, including Keanu's son: "Nor is this Keanu's only relative, his own son . . . , aged about 23, and his first cousin . . . on his mother's side, are both lepers, and reside at the Leper Settlement. [His son] has been a leper since 1873, leaving school in that year on account of the disease. Keanu's brother-in-law . . . died a tubercular leper at Kalawao, in 1885, and his (Keanu's) mother . . . was a hunchback."[54] The report identifies Keanu as both a prisoner and a patient, on the one hand indicating the ways these discussions nearly always depend on Keanu's status as a "criminal" patient and, on the other, rhetorically evoking in readers the sentimental tropes of benevolent humanism.

Even though there were many supporters among the medical community, Arning had several critics as well. Many such discussions occurred in print, not only in medical journals but also in popular literary magazines such as *Cosmopolitan*.[55] Within the first three years of the inoculation, for example, H. P. Wright published the 1888 article "The Inoculability of Leprosy" in the *British Medical Journal*. In this essay, Wright fiercely defends the reputation of Arning as a humanitarian and advocate for Hawaiian people afflicted with Hansen's disease. He ultimately used the journal to criticize Arning's detractors, stating:

> Sir,—Allow me to say a few words in defense of Dr. Arning. In England and on the Continent he has been severely blamed for inoculating Keanu, an Hawaiian, with leprosy. Surely such an attack is most unjust. This able physician is world-known for his long and skilful labour in behalf of the leper. . . . And what is the return he gets for this faithful devotion to his profession? He is publicly accused of cruelty and heartlessness for inoculating with leprosy a condemned murderer, who, to save his life, submitted willingly and gladly to the experiment.[56]

This defense of Arning, his work, and his place as a humanitarian presents a moral claim by situating the doctor as the benevolent savior and Keanu as the desperate "condemned murderer." While Arning was motivated by a desire to advance his career, H. P. Wright insists that he should be perceived as a heroic crusader. At the same time, Wright's position situates Keanu as a figure deserving to be killed—a cunning man who "save[s] his life" by opportunistically taking advantage of Arning's well-known humanitarian efforts "in behalf of the leper."

In the remainder of his article, Wright moves from his defense of Arning and the "unjust" attacks on the benevolent doctor to a peculiar speculative commentary about what Keanu might have said in this moment of consent, indexing for this discussion an important display of how Keanu's personhood emerged in print culture. Determined to show that Keanu possessed a self that was legible to his readers, he imagines Keanu's thought process, enabling Wright to speak not only for but also literally in place of the former. Wright lauded Arning's work and, of course, was not alone in his public praise of utilizing racialized, colonial, and especially criminalized subjects like Keanu for such experiments. What Wright's work demonstrates is not simply a sense of ownership and power over the thoughts and intentions of Keanu but also the production of a subject. Anthony Bogues, drawing on Michel Foucault, notes that such forms of imperial power "could not be exercised 'without knowing the inside of people's minds, without exploring their souls, without making them reveal their innermost secrets. It implies a knowledge of the conscience and an ability to direct it.'"[57] In this framing, the power to know and shape conscience became a form of power that sought to control and maintain colonial rule at the ideological level, a "drive to capture [a colonial subject's] desire and reshape it."[58] This key distinction depends on a visible shift that makes and remakes the "private intentions" of Keanu available for public inspection and consumption. Wright continued in his defense of Arning:

> Suppose for a moment, that Keanu had reasoned thus: "I readily submit to inoculation with leprosy, not only because I shall save myself from immediate death, but also for a higher reason. I have killed one man, and deep is my sorrow; should I by this inoculation become a leper, such a result may tend to save the lives of many." How far such thoughts were in the mind of Keanu we cannot say, most likely they were not there at all; but this we can say, the great benefits arising

from such a result were well in the mind of Dr. Arning, who simply carried out a compact made between Keanu and the State. The State, which could take life for the terror of evil doers, could also grant life in order to stay, if possible, in some degree, the advance of the most terrible disease that tortures man.[59]

The "private" is revealed here as the intimate knowing of Keanu's mind, soul, and "innermost secrets," serving to produce and reimagine Keanu as, at once, rational and irrational, selfless and criminal, savage and civilized, and, ultimately, free and unfree. To put this another way, Wright's speculation works to create a liberal, autonomous subject whose criminal subject position (as a prisoner) denies sovereignty over his own life but offers control enough over his own body to consent to Arning's experiments for "a higher reason" and for the benefit of Wright's narrow understanding of humanity. In Wright's speculative account of Keanu's thoughts, Keanu is made to speak his consent in a way that makes legible medical science while at the same time subsuming medical violence. To "suppose for a moment, that Keanu had reasoned thus" registers the degree to which this public conversation unfolded around Keanu, focusing most on articulating an unsettling subjectivity based in guilt and criminality. Wright's imagined confession places new value onto this criminal figure to engage the "higher reason" of both scientific enlightenment and Wright's own understanding of Christian morality. Aware of those tensions around human experimentation—reminded, perhaps, by Arning's critics—Wright deploys a logic that situates Keanu as deserving to be killed. When Wright follows with the statement, "how far such thoughts were in the mind of Keanu we cannot say, most likely they were not there at all," it illustrates how white possession manifested at this moment and structured an organizing principle of empire, and at the same time intersected with discourses of benevolence and charity. Arning and a host of others were emboldened to literally speak for Keanu, further stabilizing the conditions for Wright's explicit move to, in the same sentence, imagine and then immediately dismiss Keanu's thought processes. Wright concludes:

Dr. Arning, in a letter received by me a few days ago (December 3rd), gives the following important particulars, and asks a very reason-

able question: "The experiment was performed after mature delib-
eration, and on the authority of the advisers of the Crown and the
Privy Council of State; influential foreigners, laymen, and learned
judges reporting in committee on the subject. It was done with the
condemned criminal's written consent, and with all due care and
exactness as to really advance our knowledge of the obscure disease.
Will it not stand as having been done in the interests, not against the
laws, of humanity?"[60]

The shifting value of Keanu's life and body in this text—legally and in-
stitutionally devalued as a prisoner sentenced to death, yet extremely
valuable as a medical subject—points to a logic of exchange that produces the conditions of possibility for white supremacist science and
racial governmentality to occur publicly and relatively unchallenged
within these venues, for "advanc[ing] our knowledge of the obscure
disease."[61] Wright's quoting of Arning's "reasonable question" demonstrates how attuned the actors were to the ways settler-colonial medicine and various state mechanisms structured Keanu's commuted sentence, ultimately allowing for systematic reproduction of the conditions
of impossibility for control over one's own racially marked body.

Colonial histories in Hawai'i and Keanu's own complex subject position demonstrate how formations of a racialized, colonized, criminalized figure, and the public debates surrounding this case, were intimately tied to the conditions of impossibility for consent that were
manufactured by settler-colonial public health forces. When reading these archives against themselves, the emergence of the figure of
Keanu ought to be situated at the intersections of the long histories of
Hawaiian sovereignty movements and resistance to conditions of colonialism. The medical archive in this context emerges not as a static
collection of given facts produced by official recorded histories about
Hawai'i but rather as sites of knowledge production to be read as ways
to know a narrative of colonization that "attest[s] to its contradictions,
and yield[s] its critique."[62] This chapter turns to these archives to locate
where the producers of these kinds of knowledge, fictions, and narratives erect their subject; at the same time, it relies on these archives as
the producers of a criminal subject in order to open up a theoretical
space to read those documents against themselves, moving beyond the
meanings and the logics of empire.

Reading Consent in the Archive of *Molokai*

"Why did you bring him here?"[63] When Father Damien asks Dr. Newman, Keanu's fictional legal executor and guardian, about their arrival on the quarantine settlement on Moloka'i, he is really asking about what the doctor intends to do with his prisoner. These characters depict the first encounter of this group in O. A. Bushnell's 1963 *Molokai,* a crucial moment in the development of the novel, after Newman receives a long-awaited approval to use a convicted man as his medical subject for experimental leprosy inoculations. In Bushnell's story, Keanu does not appear to have the slow-growing bacteria *Mycobacterium leprae* (Hansen's disease) when they arrive at Kalaupapa. What reason would a medical doctor have for bringing a healthy person—and someone who is imprisoned and sentenced to death, now a ward under the care of the Hawaiian Board of Health—to this legally designated quarantined site for people diagnosed with a contagious disease? Dr. Newman represents Edward Arning and Father Damien is the Belgian priest Heilige Damiaan van Molokai (the Saint of Molokai), who was canonized in 2009 for his work to relieve the suffering of people on Kalaupapa, left to fend for themselves, which they did. Keanu, of course, represents the Kanaka Maoli prisoner-patient known for being the raw material of that medical experiment. Bushnell chose not to change the names of Damien and Keanu, which is in part why *Molokai* has consistently been read as a historical novel, documenting a medical event layered in settler-colonial politics.

Damien's direct question to Newman, though, is interpreted differently than he intended, and the doctor instead pauses to reflect on other dilemmas preoccupying him. Rather than examine what consent to deadly experiments might mean for an incarcerated person, convicted for murder and awaiting execution, Newman's thoughts wander to the problem of keeping Keanu an untainted subject for his scientific experiments. Newman, internally, reflects:

> This was a great question, as it was the great weakness, in my whole plan. How was I going to keep Keanu away from all contact with lepers, while he was set down in the midst of one of the most dismaying concentrations of lepers in the whole world? How was I going to keep him a prisoner, in a prison without walls, and at the same time leave him a free man, in spirit and in body? A free man? He was an animal,

wild and untamed. I did not need to look at him, lying sleek upon smooth rock beyond Father Damien, to know that he was like some jungle cat taking his ease in this moment of respite, but ready to spring, to run, to hunt, perhaps even to kill, when he felt the instinct rise in him again. To cage him would be to kill him; and while I felt no special affection for him, or any compulsion to spare him the caged panther's long pining and slow dying, neither did I want to jeopardize the success of my experiment upon him.[64]

Newman's thoughts are constructed, not too subtly, as the critique of a dominant scientific outlook that dehumanizes through racial logics. Having access to the doctor's intimate thoughts undoes easy identifications between reader and character, while the rational scientist follows his thoughts to their unthinkable conclusions. Keanu, Newman concludes, is not imaginable as human. Instead he becomes an animal in the doctor's instrumental mind, and therefore unnecessarily imagined within a liberal humanist tradition. Posing "A free man?" not as a statement but a question, Newman signals tropes of colonial domination, as well as a dismissive misapplication of the category "human" to a non-human subject. Throughout, Bushnell writes Newman's interiority as an ongoing dialogue that delineates human from nonhuman, as when earlier in the novel he describes Keanu as "not even a man" but "a superlatively handsome animal—exactly the animal I needed."[65] Damien's initial question, in fact—"Why did you bring him here?"—inaugurates Newman's meditation on the practical logistics of the experiment. How is it possible to keep Keanu an untainted test subject in order not to jeopardize the scientific experiment? Readers might more easily grasp the operation of scientific logic and methodology as both the strange yet familiar trope of dehumanization under multiple carceral and scientific gazes. As a tortured scientist committed to his research, that familiar humanitarian discourse of the nineteenth-century progress narratives quickly collapses around who constitutes a rights-bearing, consent-giving subject and, necessarily, who does not. The logics of medical violence and subjectivity matter too for reading the archive on which the novel is based.

A reading of *Molokai* illustrates several problems about the archive made visible through cultural production. First, that a mode of distancing from this archive is crucial for registering uneasy questions about medical science and coloniality as a state-sanctioned form of racial violence. In the fictional drama of the event, thoughts on such treatment, initiated through a question by the well-known humanitarian figure Damien, are supplanted by the impossibility of Keanu being recognized as human in the first place. Newman's initial thoughts wander quickly from his mind as he finds himself contemplating the philosophical implications of the experiment—what they might reveal about more abstract notions of freedom, containment, consent, and humanness. Ultimately, the figure that emerges from a racialized conception of criminality is one undeserving of a baseline humane treatment. The "free" in Newman's question also creates tensions that move Keanu into a predatory category, "ready to spring, to run, to hunt, perhaps even to kill, when he felt the instinct rise in him again." Bushnell's deployment and interrogations of 1880s' conceptions of freedom, contract, and liberal discourses surrounding the question of value are interconnected with those that unfolded in medical journals across empires and continents in the late nineteenth century, as discussed above. The "thoughts" of Bushnell's characters mirror the actual dialogues actively imagining the thoughts of Keanu in scientific journals, written by scientists and the general public arguing about Arning subjecting him to deadly medical experiments. Damien's question, then—"Why did you bring him here?," initially grounded in bringing Keanu from a prison in Honolulu to Moloka'i's Kalawao, "a prison without walls"—presents a philosophical conclusion that Keanu was never "a free man" but was always already a dangerous animal in need of taming, domination, and caging. How to keep Keanu a prisoner and, at the same time, leave him a free man raises other questions about how this scientific event is remembered.

Literary and cultural manifestations of medical violence and criminality reorient the construction of those official narratives, framed by what some describe as colonial fantasy, because they center medical violence and settler colonialism by retelling the story of Keanu and narrate, in this case, through the historical medical archive, a kind of counternarrative to it.[66] *Molokai* disrupts narratives by presenting colonial medicine enacted not as a national discourse of public health but as a form of legitimate state violence that shores up settler claims to Hawai'i's land and resources. The figure of Keanu in the archive helped to produce a highly valuable medical subject for study, which, as discussed above, circulated in medical journals and popular magazines. That idea reached a peak as a cultural question, as opposed to a scientific one, in Bushnell's writing—particularly in *Molokai* but in other writing as well. Shedding some light on broader questions of knowledge production in the field of American studies helps to consider its relationship to imperialism and colonialism and what this means for what Brian Roberts and Michelle Stephens call a "continentally oriented (neo)colonial modernity."[67]

Indeed, using Bushnell's novel as a focal point produces meaning differently for the medical and criminal records of Keanu held at the Hawai'i State Archives. Beginning with the fictionality of the archive does two kinds of work. First, it intentionally questions how an archival telling imposes on the historical meaning of it. Bushnell's depiction raises several problems that center the contradictions that medical modernity makes possible. Those contradictions can reflect on how culture mediates logics of race, Indigeneity, and settler memory through an engagement with medical violence and the archive it constructs. Second, it raises questions about memory, the archive, and statehood, which are interconnected, even if they are not often discussed as such.

Molokai poses problems for narrating the historical documentation of the Keanu case. Newman continuously reconciles medical violence by calling attention to other forms of state-sanctioned violence: in Keanu's case, hanging for first-degree murder. Bushnell's aim in writing historical fiction is not to read the case as a product of colonial law and imperial medicine but to highlight the importance of what he calls "a high point in Hawaii's medical history." Bushnell's 1967 biography of Arning places importance on his scientific work, suggesting that Arning managed to usher in a Hawaiian medical renaissance based on superior European scientific knowledge.[68] While Bushnell's later scholarship moves critically further away from these early reflections on Arning's work and importance to science and medicine in Hawai'i, in this 1967 biographical essay Bushnell reads as balancing sharp criticism and standing as an apologist.[69] Initial medical reports on the state of leprosy by Arning come close to admiration, when Bushnell notes: "Never before in Hawaii had such words been used, because never before had such a modern medical intellect come among the physicians of Hawaii. By the standards of their day, a few of those were good doctors; a few were quacks and derelicts, flotsam and jetsam from the seven seas and the six continents; most of them were contented mediocrities. Whether good or bad, few of them would have understood much of Arning's vocabulary or of his reasoning."[70]

A professor of medical history at the University of Hawai'i at Mānoa, Bushnell balanced the issue of historical documentation and social and cultural critique in both creative and scientific venues. He wrote histories of colonialism, imperialism, and the impacts of Western disease in the Pacific Islands and Oceania, and early in his work he valued histories of U.S. and European colonialism, particularly due to what he described as innovation in colonial medicine. Literary critic Stephen Sumida draws attention to his writing style as a multicultural hybrid, noting that the multiracial and multiethnic environment of his childhood—diasporic migrations and kinships in particular—ultimately helped him develop a literary voice that Sumida compares to William Faulkner or Mark Twain. Sumida notes that a literary technique like Bushnell's "comes naturally to a writer raised in a society characterized by the coexistence of different cultures and points of view, where, too, one is aware (as Twain and Faulkner knew), that what the outside world thinks of this locale is at odds with what the local people know."[71]

Bushnell straddles a complicated understanding of local points of view, in other words, that were the central cultural discussion in literature expressed via the 1978 Talk Story conference, as well as artistic hubs, and directly present in his early literary representations of Arning and Keanu. The cultural renaissance, Paul Lyons suggests, ought to be read through the legacy of colonialism as not only a question of economic pressure but "a specter [that] is haunting Hawai'i—the specter of sovereignty."[72] Fiction, as a cultural counternarrative to stories of colonial violence, is complex in that it navigates emerging Hawaiian nationalism and sovereignty movements—particularly as responses to statehood as defined in 1959. Dean Itsuji Saranillio, discussing resistance to colonial politics of Hawai'i statehood, notes that every state has a statehood story to tell and that writing archives is part of that story.[73] It is worth asking how Bushnell's *Molokai* works to challenge the narrative conflations and associations discussed in the previous sections of this chapter. Those naturalized constructions of racialized criminality work as a response to enduring literary tradition, which culminates with writers such as James A. Michener.[74] The broader question concerning whose work might counter narratives of imperialism and settler colonialism takes center stage at the height of Bushnell's literary career. In a keynote speech at the 1978 Talk Story: Our Voices in Literature and Song—Hawaii's Ethnic American Writers' Conference, Bushnell asserts that Hawaiian locals are letting outsiders narrate for Hawaiians who they are and what they think.[75] He states: "[Hawai'i's] writers are stifled at birth. Our geniuses with words and pen never have a chance. . . . 'Outsiders,' not only from the Mainland, will be writing the novels telling us what we are and what we think. They will turn out the stuff that the rest of the world will read."[76]

Popular novelist James A. Michener made it clear that readers outside of the islands were more than willing to take his 1959 encyclopedic novel *Hawaii* as the authoritative book on Hawaiian culture, history, and social life, as arguments for statehood.[77] Published the same year that the United States claimed Hawai'i as an official state, Michener's novel seemed to stand not only for the theft of land and ongoing colonial project of the U.S. government but also as another measure of cultural imperialism that sought to reimagine the United States as a liberal multicultural project. Sumida points to the cultural stakes of Michener's ideological novel as, in fact, more sociological and data-driven than literary:

> Whatever one may have thought about the novel's literary merits and demerits, the general feeling was that it, after all, was even by its sheer mass the most and the best those small tropical islands could muster. Why should anyone try to surpass it? Or why should anyone look for older works that have told Hawaii's story with any more authenticity or imaginative flair? Hawaii's criticism of the novel— unfavorable criticism which was quite abundant—lashed Michener for factual inaccuracies or, when he told the truth, for casting our ancestors in the lurid light of scandals involving family characters closeted generations ago.[78]

Cultural production and historiography like Michener's reveal a reliance on racist and colonial tropes, narrativization of a racialized past. Along similar lines, Sumida's point is clear: works like Michener's *Hawaii* shape the dominant narratives widely available to people across the globe. This takes on particular meaning at a moment when the example of U.S. nation-building, with the official inclusion of Hawaiʻi as the fiftieth state in the union, unfolds and is constructed as yet another passive acceptance of U.S. hegemony in Hawaiʻi.[79]

Bushnell addresses specific legal and medical conversations that begin with several iterations of colonial and settler-colonial "contact" representations, including his first novel *The Return of Lono: A Novel of Captain Cook's Last Voyage* (1956). His fiction might be read as a consistent return and revaluation of colonial historiography, again written as counternarrative to historical narratives of Hawaiʻi.[80] If print culture like the *British Medical Journal* and other scientific literature discursively produced fictions of racialized subjects, naturalizing settler medicine, *Molokai* makes colonial relations explicit and central to narratives of medicine. Published just over a decade before the Talk Story conference, it restages the story of Keanu and Arning. Focusing most on narrating from the doctor's point of view (fictionalized as Dr. Newman), Bushnell resists cultural colonial frameworks that attempt to inhabit the thoughts of the historical figure of Keanu.[81] While much writing on Hawaiʻi emerges from narratives of historical romance, depicting romantic and gendered conceptions of Hawaiʻi and Oceania as pastoral lands ready for taking, Bushnell's novel presents another type of reading. Whereas the medical archive discussed earlier produces the prisoner-patient figure in order to engender the possibility of consent for the primary purpose of making a criminalized and racialized body available and valuable for medical experimentation, Bushnell's text works to disrupt that dominant narrative not by representing the events by inhabiting and then narrating from within a subaltern subjectivity—one that speaks for the prisoner-patient who, in the official recorded archive, had no record of doing so—but instead by redirecting the colonial gaze to the doctor who manifests as legitimate imperial medical violence.

To expand on Bushnell's critique of settler time and narrative in medical and scientific discourse, James A. Michener's *Hawaii* also serves as commentary on the liberal multicultural settler refrain that dominates U.S. national narratives since annexation. Each was published during and shortly after the U.S. government ushered the territory of Hawaiʻi into the United States as the fiftieth state. The synopsis of the novel, taken from the most recent edition of the book, describes how Hawaiʻi continues to designate the temporal conditions of medical modernity and the question of time regarding statehood because it points to that enduring narrative. From the 2002 edition:

> In *Hawaii,* Pulitzer Prize–winning author James Michener weaves the classic saga that brought Hawaii's epic history vividly alive to the American public on its initial publication in 1959 and continues to mesmerize today. The volcanic processes by which the Hawaiian Islands grew from the ocean floor were inconceivably slow, and the land remained untouched by man for countless centuries until, little more than a thousand years ago, Polynesian seafarers made the perilous journey across the Pacific and discovered their new home. They lived and flourished in this tropical paradise according to their ancient traditions and beliefs until, in the early nineteenth century, American missionaries arrived, bringing a new creed and a new way of life to a Stone Age society. The impact of the missionaries had only begun to be absorbed when other national groups, with equally different customs, began to migrate in great numbers to the islands. The story of modern Hawaii, and this novel, is one of how disparate peoples, struggling to keep their identity yet live with one another in harmony, ultimately joined together to build America's strong and vital fiftieth state.[82]

In relation to its continued popularity and framing in the current moment, contemporary settler memory is imagined as the creation myths of nineteenth-century American missionaries. The historical conditions of Hawai'i culminate in "modern Hawaii" as a struggle over identity and the ability for a "Stone Age society" to live "in harmony" with settlers, who simply brought "a new creed and a new way of life" to an ancient world. As scholars note, that it functioned as a cultural extension of the United States as a statehood novel helps to situate the refrain as mining the past to define the present, not as its conditions of possibility as its oppositional racial other. As settler time, the past cannot exist in the present or future, but the past represents a racialized figure of Polynesian people and the present/future represents an American nation-state that dominates in the form of the settler state. Through statehood, in other words, Hawai'i "ultimately joined together to build America's strong and vital fiftieth state," squaring the temporal development in/of 1959 that narrates a colonization as immigration, rather than dismantling, dispossessing, annexing, territorializing, and absorbing through the nomenclature of "statehood," joining a nation as the latest piece in the puzzle of liberal modernity.[83] What marks mass culture also marks what constitutes "the public" in relation to a global frame, and *Hawaii* serves as one major form of cultural imperialist imaginative work producing scientific settler logics that has a long history.

Reading *Hawaii* against Bushnell's *Molokai*, published just four years after Michener's widely read and praised novel, that tension takes on a different referent. With these discussions in mind, other connections between the progress narrative of science and medicine and the production of difference through race, criminality, and power that are the conditions of medical violence in carceral and medical spaces can be drawn. The cultural politics of medicine in the realm of what might be understood as scientific settler literature relies on the qualifier *settler* to signal those literatures structuring medicine, criminality, and the category of the human, setting a kind of imaginative stage for mapping the transits of medical violence through print culture. Medical journals and other forms of public and intimate conversations about science in colonial spaces circulate as their own political and cultural imperial narrative—what Bushnell's last book calls "the gifts of civilization."[84] Given that Bushnell took up, as a final project, a critical interrogation of imperial scientific histories, we might read this as the alterity of the scientific settler.

The publication timing of these two novels, *Hawaii* and *Molokai*, matters too. *Hawaii* was published on, and *Molokai* four years after, the finality of Hawai'i as the official fiftieth state. It also points to a moment when Native resistance movements demanded and held political and cultural sway over U.S. empire, in concert with sovereignty moments and the heightened visibility of decolonial thought across the colonized world. This cultural moment and these novels find themselves articulating their politics in radicalized contexts, working within narratives of developmental modernity, moving from the structuring tropes of literature and multiple contradictions presented in colonial imaginaries—from past to present and future, from ancient to modern. While part of this chapter outlines where those moments find cultural and political value in the production of a Western subject, and in firming up nation and citizen, it is also possible to read Bushnell's novel as a site of collapse and contradiction, one that resists development even as it deploys, generically, tools of producing the insinuation of liberal thought into governing cultural institutions. This interrogation of memory and official history is at heart speculative in that it wrestles with the present through the past historical narrative to hold the present and the future in tension—between the categories of history, memory, and futurity, allowing for something else to surface and show what the nation-state continues to mean in the present.

The Archive as Question

In 2016, the Hawai'i State Archives in Honolulu launched its 110th anniversary celebration, highlighting the institution's vast collections and long service of preservation. In a news interview publicizing the event, one archivist noted that the archive contained "an amazing diversity of history, from pre-constitutional government, the monarchy, the provisional government, the republic, the territory and the state."[85] The celebration emphasized the role of such spaces in documenting the work and histories of Hawai'i through its contested governmental life and, more importantly, affirmed its shifting responsibility to serve the larger community: "It all resides within this building and we have to take this opportunity to share it with the people." At an open house at the Hawai'i State Archives, people were invited to learn about the holdings, which included displays of Queen Lili'uokalani's marriage license and personal song book, an early draft of Abraham Lincoln's Emancipation Proclamation, a Pearl Harbor exhibit in honor of the seventy-fifth anniversary of the attack on the military naval base, and the "official" pen that President Dwight Eisenhower used to sign Hawai'i, a U.S. territory, into statehood in 1959.

Not a curated exhibit so much as a display of archival holdings, it is worth pressing on several questions that get at what meanings are produced by the space, and what it is supposed to do for the present. Archivists worked, for example, to situate the documents and artifacts for visitors as both dominant and dissenting narratives. That visitors from the community, along with scholars and researchers, were invited to sit with the contradictions housed in the building in downtown Honolulu suggests that this event sought to put some critical pressure on the conventional meaning of state archives as not only a repository of national significance but more a community resource of collective memory. Yet the narration of this event took on some familiar historical trajectories, defaulting to the times of the nation-state and the production of national identity. In the archivist's statement, moving from nineteenth-century narratives into an inevitable present marked by progress, modernity, and national futures, this story presents Hawai'i as in natural transition from monarchy to representative democracy. That temporal constitution manages a developmental story of liberal modernity—from enslavement to freedom, from colonial military occupation to U.S. territory status, and finally ending in statehood with the literal stroke of a presidential pen.

In the Introduction I noted that a conception of medical modernity shapes the very idea of who belongs and who does not around flexible notions of personhood and racial violence, implicated in the understanding of history as a series of unbroken moments propelled forward in time. When tethered to some notion of usable subjects, such as prisoners who are at the same time patients, the unfolding of that official historical narrative clings to stories of progress in service of the state and maintains a stabilized notion of a "public" and the terms of citizenship within it. A medical modernity contributes to the formations of knowledge around what is imagined in the figure of the prisoner and patient. This is important for a reconsideration of science, medicine, and criminality. Archives at the Hawai'i State Archives—specifically those pertaining to public health in the nineteenth century—unsettle this developmental narrative of medical violence that is also linked to forwarding a state imperative to manage race, Indigeneity, and criminality. I turn to fiction as the counterpoint to the implicit fictions of medical archives, moving toward the limit point of a prisoner-patient in nineteenth-century Hawai'i. As a bildungsroman of medical imaginaries structured by the inevitability of the nation-state, the incorporation of state violence conjured in the national story moves through a logics of who makes scientific progress matter for these stories, who are the conditions of it, who tells those stories, and where and what happens when narratives of progress collide with state-sanctioned violence.

A genealogy suggests that those tensions read in the context of the state archives as anxieties of historical preservation, recovery, and retrieval move as a singular, unfolding narrative. To return to the archivist's description above, what makes "an amazing diversity of history" relies on the legible line of thought and historical events leading to statehood—"from pre-constitutional government, the monarchy, the provisional government, the republic, the territory and the state." All these developmental stages are preserved within the walls of the state archives, framing those documents, as well as the buildings housing them, as emerging from the past, present, and future colonial state. The state archives provides the location to engage different kinds of questioning of historical narratives—and to do it as a question. As I discussed in the Introduction, Lisa Lowe's reflection on theoretical inquiry via recovery is useful here as well. To question under what conditions notions such as freedom and unfreedom can be examined historically "mobilizes the different valences of the term." How the retrieval of archival evidence potentially ignites "the restoration of historical presence" matters for the work of theorizing the archive as an articulation for the present. Absence and presence of representation in history is, in one sense, what the archive represents. In another, the "ontological and political sense of reparation," meaning the definitional parameters of redress and justice as ontological and political questions, signifies not only a question of historical presence but political subjectivity.[86] Lowe's elaboration on the possibility of recuperation is also represented by the "repossession of a full humanity and freedom, after its ultimate theft or obliteration," a tension that troubles notions of recovery as anchored to forms of historical analysis that locate "full humanity" within a rubric of power producing those conditions to interpret it as such.[87] This is to say that it requires reading the archive, and its conditions, against itself, so that reading the archive paradoxically is to interpret "recovery as a question, and not as an established project or tradition."[88]

Reading the Hawai'i State Archives, and reading it as a question, was prompted by my visit in 2017, just a few months before the open house. I was there searching through nineteenth-century police reports, court documents, and medical photographs, looking to recover the government files on a man named Keanu. The case was sensationalized in English-language newspapers, yet what ultimately made Keanu famous was not his crime but rather how he was made to pay for it. Again, Keanu could pay his debts to society by consenting to be the raw materials in medical experiments. The rationale, simplified, follows this line: there was a murder, a conviction, and a sentence to death, the death sentence was commuted to life in prison, and then Keanu was handed over to a scientist so that he could try to transmit Hansen's disease to him—to ultimately try to kill him. Devaluing this life as a prisoner would be revalued through scientific and humanitarian work, to advance science so that others may benefit. The act, too, brings a premodern past to the modern present, something even Bushnell acknowledges in his early scientific writing about Arning. While the doctor plays the central role in this story, there was a matrix that created the conditions for understanding Keanu as a devalued life in order to manufacture a valuable human subject available for scientific settler colonialism.[89]

The question, then, is not the spectacle of this event but the more mundane, routine articulations of state and colonial violence that fill the rooms of government buildings: boxes of court proceedings, meeting minutes, and council notes. It was the minutia that captures a profound discussion of the ways to best manage people living and working in Hawai'i: budgets on medical facilities for quarantine sites and patient counts, piles of files filled with images visually documenting various stages of Hansen's disease through scientific settler-colonial gazes. The problem of "looking" at certain archives—particularly at medical violence in these visual archives, photographs, measurements, and meditations on bodies—turned into problems of registering the archival traces never intended to be seen, considered, or thought about outside of medical and scientific worlds and considering how those traces were captured and then exceeded the parameters they inhabited over decades. It is necessary, in other words, to consider what conditions produced their value as documents in need of preservation and, ultimately, to examine what this means for the preservation of colonial and, more broadly, contested histories of medical and state violence. Questioning recovery—and what gets to be considered recoverable and for what purposes—places the discussion of archives in another realm.

The Hawai'i State Archives' creation under statute in 1905 allowed for its opening in 1906. Following the 1893 illegal overthrow of the monarchy, the installation of the provisional government, the 1898 annexation, and the establishment as a territory with the Hawaiian Organic Act of 1900, the time of this moment has been critically examined by historians like Osorio.[90] The open house in 2016 was prompted by American Archives Month, established by the National Archives in Washington, D.C., to raise awareness about the value of archives and archivists across the United States. The origins of the Hawai'i State

Archives came out of a desire to protect, as a new territory of the United States, what the colonial governmental administrators in nineteenth-century Hawaiʻi knew to be important materials of the islands located there rather than in Washington, D.C. "Shortly after annexation," Governor George Carter's *Report of the Governor of the Territory of Hawaii to the Secretary of the Interior 1905* explains, "the Chief of the United States Bureau of Archives came to Hawaii to look up these documents with a view to have them transferred to Washington, but finally consented to leave them in the Territory, on assurance that every effort would be made to secure a fireproof hall for their preservation, particularly as it was claimed that their relations to land titles was too important to have them leave the Territory."[91]

Archivist Jason Horn, in a 1953 summation of the history of the Hawaiʻi State Archives leading up to statehood, notes: "This transition was opposed by Hawaiian leaders"—that is, political and business leaders who were influential in managing the Territory of Hawaiʻi, which likely included first territorial governor Sanford B. Dole—"particularly on the grounds that the relation of the records to land titles was too important for the records to leave Hawaii."[92] Other streams of appropriated funding from this mandate allowed for creating an archives board, which would ultimately assist in consolidating and maintaining bureaucratic power over the new territory: "Meanwhile," Horn continues, "by another act of the legislature approved April 3, 1905, the broad organization and functions of the Archives of Hawaii were established.... It provides for the establishment of a three-man Board of Commissioners of Public Archives."[93] Members of this newly established first board were also those highest in colonial offices and positions, including administrative member (under both King Kalākaua's and Queen Liliʻuokalani's rule and later under the provisional government) Alatau Tamchiboulac Atkinson; professor and college president William DeWitt Alexander, a Hawaiian-born son of missionaries from Kentucky and influential writer on Hawaiian history and language; and lawyer and territory trust officer Albert Francis Judd Jr., grandson of U.S. missionary and adviser to King Kamehameha Gerrit Parmele Judd and son of Justice Albert Francis Judd, who sentenced Keanu to death in 1884.[94] The board appointed Robert Colfax Lydecker as its first archives secretary on May 10, 1905.

Indeed, the general sentiment surrounding the creation of the archive was explicitly colonial, deploying the same kinds of civilizing language found in early missionary writings and the same that underpins future state projects, such as James Michener's *Hawaii*. That is, the praise for the construction of the state archive facilities is reflected in the governor's report to the secretary of the interior in 1905, which states: "It is a matter of congratulations to the Territory that the work of caring for and preserving these valuable documents, tracing as they do the history of Hawaii from the darkness of heathenism, through the sunlight of Christianity, and down to the present time, is at last to be undertaken in a manner that will insure their future preservation. It is a duty that has been too long neglected and one that the country owes to posterity."[95] On the preservation of James Cook's materials, which was initiated in 1928 by librarian of the archives Albert Pierce Taylor, who early on worked with Hawaii Supreme Court Justice and contributing author of the 1900 Hawaiian Organic Act Walter F. Frear, Horn writes: "The Captain Cook memorial collection comprises a major part of the Archives' holdings of eighteenth-century material, which increase a little each year by purchases financed by the Captain Cook memorial fund. This fund was created during the 1928 celebration of the discovery of the Hawaiian Islands 150 years before by Captain Cook." Taylor, then state archivist, was a member of the Captain Cook Sesquicentennial Commission, which was responsible for staging the celebration and linking it to the state archives and their holdings. The Captain Cook Memorial Collection sought to acquire vast materials to bridge the gap between the "discovery of the islands and the inauguration of the monarchy." As Horn puts it: "Enabling legislation permits the Archivist to use the fund to collect documents relating to Cook's life or connected with his discovery of the islands. The collection includes photostats and other copies of logs, journals, diaries of members of the Cook and Vancouver expeditions to Hawaii."[96]

The narration of the archive as "such an amazing diversity of history" presses on the very logic of liberalism that produces, and then subsumes, the contestation that is not in question as the dominant narrative. What constituted a need to preserve records? And how might it continue to imagine, against an aggressive disavowal of state violence through inevitable formations of empire, militarism, and the nation-state, a different kind of narrative?[97]

CHAPTER 2

Memory, Memoir, and the Carville Leprosarium

The official version is in everybody's mouth. . . .
This is what happened; this is how it was.

—MICHELLE CLIFF, *FREE ENTERPRISE:
A NOVEL OF MARY ELLEN PLEASANT*

This chapter examines the site of Carville as a field of medical violence that contends with discourses of an emerging public health nationalism. As Hansen's disease shaped the formations of race in Hawai'i as science and U.S. military occupation to U.S. territorial governance, firmer lines are put forth to argue that Pacific Islands and the U.S. South need to be articulated as two different nationally symbolic sites surrounding public health. A white subject emerged from Hawai'i and significant spaces for colonial medicine. Following the above discussion in Congress regarding the federal funding for medical and scientific resources at Kalaupapa, Moloka'i, what the national discourse imagined for the future of U.S. public health was something very different. Racialized patients, residents, and others remember Carville, particularly in relation to its histories of race and settler colonialism, though certainly few regard it explicitly as such. By reading Michelle Cliff's novel *Free Enterprise,* memoirs by Stanley Stein and José P. Ramirez Jr., and the archive of patient Josefina "Joey" Guerrero, whose public persona was a Filipina resistance fighter supporting U.S. soldiers in Manila under Japanese occupation, this chapter suggests that the insertion of race and memory into this archive—whether via nonfictional memoir, through documentary traces, or fictional engagement—invites rethinking the logics of race and property within it. This chapter also examines the entwined racialization of memory, politics, and public health as the implications of Hansen's disease for the United States as they unfold in the space of Carville, Louisiana.

In 1932, during a congressional hearing to discuss the need for federal aid to maintain Hawai'i's medical infrastructure for Hansen's disease treatment, Republican delegate of the territory of Hawai'i Victor S. Kaleoaloha Houston proposed H.R. Bill 306 to address underfunded patient care. The Kalaupapa settlement on Moloka'i and the Kalihi Receiving Hospital in Honolulu were a topic of debate, as was the future of living conditions of more than six hundred patients residing within those spaces. The proposal requested U.S. appropriations for maintaining "the care of lepers in the Territory of Hawaii," and the exchange that followed between Houston and microbiologist Dr. McCoy bears witness to a ghostly obsession with situating what race means for understanding Hansen's disease.[1] How to fund and maintain the many research possibilities circulating across the globe remained a looming question for the U.S. government in navigating racial capital and settler states.[2] In particular, human research was a major focus, though also a minor obstacle, given small attention to critical discussions about criminality and patient consent. Quoting at length Houston and McCoy's reference to Keanu (discussed in the previous chapter) points to much larger questions here:

> Mr. Houston. I suppose you recollect having heard of the case in Hawaii under the kingdom, of the criminal who was given the choice of submitting to capital punishment or to a test for leprosy. He had been adjudged guilty of a capital punishment crime, and he was inoculated, as I understand, with some of the material on his breast, and he never developed leprosy subsequently; is that true?
>
> Doctor McCoy. Well, if you and I are thinking of the same man, Keanu, the subject of the test did develop leprosy two years after the operation. He died on Molokai. But that is the solitary successful—if you call it successful—example of transference of leprosy by the experimental method. In discussing that case I always feel that I must explain that Keanu, of course, was a Hawaiian, and at that time something like 2 or 3 per cent of adult Hawaiians were infected with leprosy, so that there is a chance that he might have become a leper without inoculation; on the other hand, the first sign of leprosy was

noted at the point of inoculation, and I am disposed to regard it as a valid example of experimental inoculation.[3]

Houston was a high-ranking U.S. Navy officer before serving as a delegate from 1927 to 1933, and he was known for supporting the territory through the development of commerce. He navigated Hawai'i–U.S. relations as the son of a U.S. Navy admiral from Pennsylvania and as a descendant of a prominent Kānaka 'Ōiwi family from Honolulu.[4] The H.R. 306 proposal ultimately put up for debate the stakes in defining Hawai'i's right, as a U.S. territory, to federal funding and other state resources, anchoring those arguments by looking to the Department of Justice (DOJ)—specifically the appropriations designated for ad hoc prisons in U.S. territories, where the United States would be charged with "the care of Federal prisoners in such areas or places where there are not Federal institutions for their disposal."[5] To identify a precedent for funding and DOJ's management of jails and prisons in colonial and territorial legal contexts provided Houston one site for resources.

After two days of discussions about delegating funds to Hawai'i, however, members of Congress began formulating objections, signaling a distinct discourse of colonial management. Why had the Philippines, as another territory of the United States, not requested funding from the federal government to address how to deal with the spread of Hansen's disease there?[6] Perhaps race and "tropical climates" should be considered further as the determining factor for why the disease had spread so dramatically.[7] Would not continuing quarantine measures—meaning police arrest, coercion, or encouragement to self-surrender—be more appropriate in those spaces, rather than providing additional funding to support medical care facilities such as hospitals?[8] What would federal funding provide the territories in the Pacific Islands as opposed to people living on the U.S. Mainland?[9] More specifically, why should Hawai'i receive federal aid when the Carville facility seemed to thrive? The National Leprosarium at Carville in Louisiana, while managed under the United States Public Health Services, seemed to be a different kind of medicalized space than the ones that emerged in Hawai'i under the more coercive colonial Act to Prevent the Spread of Leprosy. In other words, the Carville Leprosarium began to represent to policy makers and lawmakers not just an investment in medical knowledge developed in research facilities but also the possibility to treat groups of people voluntarily and with their consent. This shift to being concerned with both the medical knowledge and the quarantined patient from which knowledge was produced was framed as a budgetary and practical issue. Houston questions, though indirectly, what allows public health officials to classify a medical space as a research center and what makes it a space (i.e., a hospital) that should be concerned primarily with patient care and well-being: "There is only one Federal leprosy institution in the United States" that does both, Houston notes, "and that is at Carville, La."[10]

Arriving late to the hearing, eugenicist Congressman Albert Johnson snidely remarked on what he perceived to be Houston's ulterior motives—that is, assistance and resources for "non-white" people infecting the national polity: "I think there is something else in the minds of the people of Hawaii. They want local self-government with plenty of Federal aid. [Laughter.]"[11] Houston's supposed Hawaiian-ness provided a familiar framing for foreignness as an ongoing threat to white people. Albert Johnson—coauthor, with Senator David Reed, of the 1924 anti-immigrant, antilabor Johnson-Reed Act, passed only eight years before—was also president of the Eugenics Research Association from 1923 to 1924, an organization that pushed for public policy based on eugenics. Johnson, however, was a longtime congressional advocate for the eugenics movement and its implementation into U.S. immigration law.[12] His views guided his political moves to create stringent limits and quotas on supposedly undesirable immigrants that were not originating from northern and western European nations, as he argued very publicly through his newspapers (he owned the *Grays Harbor Washingtonian,* based in Hoquiam, Washington) and on a political platform that northern and western Europeans were more intelligent, democratic, and more readily assimilable into the United States. The nature of these discussions as xenophobic, racist, and anti-immigrant surface throughout the 1932 congressional hearings. But the most explicit back-and-forth between the medical experts on leprosy in Hawai'i and Carville during the committee hearings gets at the underlying logics of race and disease not as a global or even a colonial concern but as a specific issue for the United States to handle. Regarding Carville specifically, the chairman prompted a debate about how they might press scientists to define it as such:

CHAIRMAN: Leprosy is a national problem.

MR. DOUGLASS. Yes. I do not doubt that.

MR. PARSONS. With reference to the 350 or so we have at Carville, what is the nationality of those people? Are they Caucasians—our own native people?

DOCTOR MCCOY. Very largely our own people: very largely white stock. Those patients largely come from the Gulf coast.

MR. PARSONS. In your observation there is nothing with reference to climatic conditions or of the races to indicate anything either way with reference to leprosy?

DOCTOR MCCOY. I would qualify that a little. Climatic conditions, or geographical conditions rather than climatic, apparently control the communicability of the disease. I can not tell you why they do, but that is a hard, cold fact. The patients are scathed from all States, from practically all States. Louisiana, of course, furnishes the largest single number at Carville, 98; Texas, 34. Those two furnish the largest numbers. The majority are from the Gulf Coast States. There always are a few Chinese and Japanese at Carville; and there were 11 Hawaiians in the last census in Carville.

MR. FINLEY. How many negroes are there?

DOCTOR MCCOY. A very considerable number. I do not have the figures here as to race, but there are always a lot of negroes in Carville, perhaps 75 or a hundred....

THE CHAIRMAN. Are there any Mexicans down there?

DOCTOR MCCOY. Some Mexicans; yes.

DOCTOR CUMMING. The reason there are not more foreigners now is that the Immigration Service has been more active, and where we have found aliens we have turned them over, and they are sent out of the country.

MR. DOWELL. Has any study been made by you or others with reference to race, different races contracting this disease? Does the race have anything to do with it, in other words?[13]

With testimony as the driver of the hearing, they drew lines to demarcate the Gulf Coast threshold of white patients—"Caucasians—our own native people"—against nonwhite, foreign, and "other" people who may be positioned as the cause, if not the transmitter, of the disease. As such, the debate followed to manage a question of national security under the guise of national health protection. While Johnson's efforts to protect white people through immigration policies of the 1920s had already been widely accepted in Congress—meaning both the protection of economic and political supremacy for white people in the United States and protection from undesirable people and customs—xenophobia and national security permeated all conversations about public health, as we see in regard to Carville.[14]

While the hearings discussed above are just one example of how the official versions of public health reconcile medical violence, the debates about public safety—as well as those about territorial management— affected how laws and policy were perceived, including those that followed as Carville became a center for research. What was at stake had to do with understanding the state's authority to surveil, inspect, and manage the bodies of citizens and noncitizens—to "identify certain individuals as threats to the public health, and confine them within specialized institutions," as Michelle Moran aptly puts it.[15] The management of race and disease in Louisiana at the turn of the century also works out colonial logics around Hawai'i.[16] Medical practices between doctors and administrators in Hawai'i and the U.S. South not only replicate in the South medical knowledge developed in the territory but negotiated other particularities that included racialized and gendered policies, writing through medicine, and general racial assumptions that were mapped onto Native Hawaiians. Racial and colonial narratives shift and transform as the spaces and places of public health attempt to control national narratives. In the case of Hawai'i, that language was dominated by long-standing colonial imaginaries that represent Hawaiians as promiscuous or ignorant, particularly as health officials reflected on how patients, residents, and family members resisted forms of scientific and medical racialism.[17]

Michelle T. Moran's *Colonizing Leprosy: Imperialism and the Politics of Public Health in the United States* draws contentions between the colonial underpinnings that dialectically produce public health in Hawai'i and Louisiana. Moran argues that to read in isolation or to take analyses out of their imperial contexts misses the enduring dialogue occurring between Mainland and colonial spaces. I would push this insight further: carceral and settler-colonial logics of those medical institutions are not overlooked symptoms, missed because the wrong lens has been applied to them. They might instead be approached as constitutive. Where the overlooked (unseen, illegible, ignored) framework suggests things left out, what occurs instead is a process that enfolds violence into its progress narrative. The dialogue in medical journals and public health policy shaped how bodies were medicalized through racialized and gendered lenses across Oceania and the Pacific Archipelago, the Caribbean, Europe, Africa, Asia, and, specific for this conversation, the United States.[18] Also significant, however, is that those practices find traction, provide language for, and produce conditions of the unfolding discussions about Carville and across other medical spaces. Regarding colonial practices transported to public health institutions within U.S. borders, the establishment of medical facilities in Hawai'i and Louisiana researching and treating Hansen's disease had produced the perception that public health facilities and infrastructures were crucial and needed to be funded. Tracing those financial discussions in culture and in archives leads to other questions about the racialization of bodies through disease.

In Carville, however, health officials implemented restrictive policies and mandated that "patients follow the dictates of the modern medical institution" differently than at Kalaupapa.[19] The dialectical shift of knowledge from the Pacific, the Philippines, the Caribbean, and beyond, in other words, laid a foundation for a Louisiana counterpart. It was ultimately patients at Carville "who acted as ideal test subjects in medical research" because the evolution of public health in the United States emerges from fortifying national borders and regulating immigration under both imperial and nativist (eugenicist) frameworks.[20] Thus, Warwick Anderson, in a retooling of José David Saldívar's writing on the U.S.–Mexico borderlands, describes "the colonial laboratories" of the Philippines, Puerto Rico, and Hawai'i as its own colonial form of scientific borderlands, "where many 'experts' were experimenting with various national bodies." Anderson takes this dynamic exchange of scientific discourse across borders and oceans as a starting point:

> The medical doctors and bureaucrats I write about were itinerants, with a global view of things that historians, so preoccupied with the local and constrained by nation or region, are only now coming to appreciate. In a generally uncritical, unreflective way, these colonial technicians were prepared to find the modern in the colony, the colonial in the metropole. In this case, the traffic between the

United States and the Philippines, the Pacific crossings, enables us to recognize that colonial technologies of rule could also be used to develop the "nation" and its various disciplines in both locations. The experience of empire allowed American scientists and physicians to bring many colonial bureaucratic practices—and even a new sense of themselves—back to urban health departments in the United States and elsewhere between 1910 and 1920.[21]

As my reading of the debates in hearings suggests, there were great differences in how those spaces were constructed and maintained based on national narratives about race, citizenship, and imperial fantasy, and only after medical officials made strides at Carville treating patients with experimental sulfone drugs for several years in the late 1940s did those treatments become available to patients in Hawaiʻi. Indeed, what made this possible was patient activism in Kalaupapa and Kalawao on Molokaʻi, which prompted, as Neel Ahuja notes, "new possibilities for reframing the history and struggles of Hawaiian patients impacted by the segregation order."[22] While none of these scholarly accounts considers the cultural, political, and social significance of Edward Arning's experimental inoculations on Keanu in the 1880s, which, in part, can be read into the medical triumph narrative that culminates at Carville in the mid- and late twentieth century, the important insights of a global dialogue across geographical locations are clear. Though ideologies of white supremacy and colonial context shaped each place in significantly different ways, the medical institutions across locations were in close contact at every stage and developed in conversation with one another. With those insights in mind, the remainder of this chapter examines memory and memory work of writers and patients thinking through the meaning of Carville and how it has contributed to imagining and reconstructing the archival memory of Carville as a site of contestation.

Memory and Archive

In the chapter entitled "U.S. Public Health Service Station #66" of Michelle Cliff's 1993 novel *Free Enterprise,* a snarky narrator reflects on the discourse of leprosy as "a disease peculiar to humans" and, especially, the anxiety-driven research that emerges not from its contagiousness but rather its origins.[23] Parodying a voice of medical authority, the narrator insists that no one "knows exactly how, or when, leprosy entered the United States," but then speculates: "It is safe to guess that the disease flourishes among the darker races. When you read the literature on leprosy, also known as Hansen's disease, the search for point of entry into the U.S.A. appears as crucial as the search for the cure, vaccine." Not directly naming it, the chapter goes on to bring attention to the colonial histories of medical surveillance and to reconcile racial anxiety in the United States. At the same time, it highlights settler-colonial and imperial identities with what Ahuja calls dread life—or the state's negotiation of contagious, criminalized bodies as impetus for bolstering public security.[24] Cliff's poetry, novels, and essays put such official histories under a kind of poetic scrutiny, a tension noted in a 1994 interview about what she sought to work out in her writing: "I started out as an historian; I did my graduate work in history. I've always been struck by the misrepresentation of history and have tried to correct received versions of history, especially the history of resistance."[25] While Cliff regularly describes *Free Enterprise* as a "whole novel . . . about resistance," centering stories of forgotten people from across the globe who define their own relationships to dispossession, she also extends a critical lens "to re-vision history" to that of place, time, and memory. Specifically, Cliff sets out to reimagine how people inhabited the Leprosarium in Carville, as prisoner-patients who have resisted, even as it is remembered as something else.[26] In "Oral Histories," the chapter following "U.S. Public Health Service Station #66," Cliff depicts a more playful conversation between her protagonist Annie Christmas and a group of incarcerated patients. Sneaking into the grounds the same way people snuck out—through a hole in the fence—Christmas communes with the group: "Some among them had a burning desire to escape. Some did not. Some had made their peace with the place, and their affliction; others not so." The narrator then introduces them all as a motley group with something in common: they find value in each other as they navigate their medicalized incarceration through story and remembering. "There were stories about a flatboat tied and hidden among the reeds at the riverside. There were stories of one man in particular, labeled incorrigible, trying to make his way back to Hawai'i, where his people were."[27]

As a whole, *Free Enterprise* complicates the figure of John Brown in the story of Black freedom; indeed, Brown serves as a minor character in the story, as Cliff draws specific attention to the gendered dynamics in the ways both official and radical histories rely heavily on the heroic progress narratives of freedom and liberation. The novel has been examined in its relation to postcolonial and feminist theory and its attempts to interrogate the histories of abolition—particularly as it is structured by the mythologies surrounding John Brown—by centering instead the stories of two Black women, Mary Ellen Pleasant and Annie Christmas. Pleasant's role in raising funds in San Francisco as an entrepreneur (the play of the book's title, *Free Enterprise,* hints at this) to support what is ultimately understood as Brown's rebellion has been illegible until feminist, decolonial accounts have worked to recover it. As the narrator puts it: "When the smoke cleared the name officially attached to the deed was John Brown. Who has ever heard of Annie Christmas, Mary Shadd Carey, Mary Ellen Pleasant?"[28] And as *Free Enterprise* centers the radical work of Black women, it also understands revisioning history to mean broadening what liberation is, and for whom. Cliff identifies resistance in this way not in grand liberation narratives but rather in the mundane, be it in the forms of sharing stories with strangers, remembering and reconstituting kinships, and locating more robust forms of struggle.[29]

The "incorrigible" man from Hawai'i, a descendant of "feathered kings, so he said," shows the group a scrimshawed human thigh bone, which had carved into it "the last moments of Captain Cook." Made by his great-grandfather as a gift to his great-grandson, the man tells the "tale of the scrimshaw to some of his fellow lepers, in his great-grandfather's words, one humid Saturday night as the rest of the [Carville] colony watches a tennis tournament under newly installed lights."[30] In the voice of his great-grandfather, who witnessed the first arrival of James Cook and his crew, the group is momentarily transported in time: "When I first laid eyes on them they were sitting on the beach—and I don't intend this as an apology—I want to tell you what happened. They were sitting on the beach. Their longboats, plain of decoration, unlike our own canoes—those of the Maori, Mayan, Arawak, Carib, Aztec, Ashanti, Yoruba, Samoan, Inuit—all the people we met on the seas—their longboats were pulled up against the shore, which they called, we found out later, the Strand. This comforted them, it seemed, and satisfied their desire to christen everything anew—even us."[31]

Carville in Cliff's depictions represents both sites of foreclosure and possibility. First, that the construction of memory at Carville reveals not the linear temporalities of the nation, specifically the U.S. Public Health Services, but rather its unfinished work as a racialized imperial project. When the incorrigible man from Hawaiʻi tells his great-grandfather's encounter with Cook as a pivotal moment of colonial history, he does so by inhabiting the memory of his kin rather than by narrating the events as they come down, so to speak, from above. That is, like Brown in the story of Mary Ellen Pleasant and Annie Christmas, Cook is a minor character who happens to show up. In the case of Cook, more happenstance and out of place than the imperial icon that history remembers him to be: "Their clothes were as plain as their boats. And heavy. It was as if they hadn't planned on ending up here, under our blazing sun. As if, as they made their progress across the world, the sun would be the one they knew from home. Their own sun would follow them, light their way, make them comfortable."[32]

What is found in *Free Enterprise,* in other words, is a displacement of settler time, similar to what Mark Rifkin describes as a "deferring [of] juridical time," a suspension of the problem of locating Indigenous experience within settler governance, frameworks, and lifeworlds.[33] Second, that by looking to memory work about Carville we find a genre of narrative—such as memoir, but also the illness narrative in news media, politics, and public health and security—that points to a dialectic of racial liberalism and consent emerging from medical violence. Cliff explores the very collision between the official narratives and patient memory at Carville, depicting dialogues that survive as the undercurrents of that space. I find Cliff's literary descriptions of history particularly apt to engage with the twentieth-century memory work of this chapter, such as memoir and archiving, because it is the official version in everyone's mouth that *Archiving Medical Violence* seeks to interrogate, especially as it is constructed around a notion of sanctioned medical violence. While many have contended with the invisible histories surrounding not just Carville but Louisiana's Indigenous histories and histories of plantation slavery, this chapter proposes Carville as a useful site of historical struggle.[34]

The centering of Carville as an anchor for unsteady histories of race and criminality of the global U.S. South—a space where people and histories from across lands and oceans converge—is no accident.

Home to the National Hansen's Disease Museum and Archive, the grounds of Carville hold the memories of people who were quarantined, as well as the institutional history of the space, often beginning with the story of the Sisters of Charity caring for Hansen's disease patients taken out of New Orleans. Those patients were housed in the former slave plantation with its modest origins, beginning in a makeshift hospital made from the preexisting slave quarters—the only usable structure found there on the plantation, which was abandoned during Reconstruction. It is also where patient residents lived complex lives while under quarantine. It occupies the ancestral lands of the Houma people, whose descendants reside currently as the United Houma Nation in Terrebonne and Lafourche Parishes, in the southern part of present-day Louisiana. The location of the leprosarium and museum was formerly the site of a ruined sugar plantation in the Reconstruction era. It was an ad hoc hospital for quarantined Hansen's disease patients in 1894, later transformed under the United States Public Health Services into the National Leprosarium and research center in 1921. It remained a home for patient residents even while the U.S. government reclaimed the space as an overflow federal prison in 1991. It was placed on the National Register of Historic Places under the National Park Services in 1992 and was then a headquarters for the National Guard during Hurricane Katrina in 2005, which it remains today. The year 1995 inaugurated the National Hansen's Disease Museum. The Gillis W. Long Center at Carville—housed in the original plantation mansion, designed between 1857 and 1859 by the well-known plantation architect Henry Howard—is one of seven National Guard military installations in Louisiana. Under the Department of Health and Human Services and Health Resources and Services Administration, the National Hansen's Disease Museum holds paraphernalia, medical records, and the Stanley Stein, alias for Sidney Levyson (1899–1967), Archive, which was organized and filed by Stein while he lived as a patient after he was brought to Carville for treatment in 1931.[35]

A kind of palimpsest, Carville appeals to the transformative idea that is U.S. settler colonialism. It attracts tourists and researchers from across the United States and beyond because it holds over a century of memories, archives, and stories, while at the same time subsuming those very histories through its tourism and narration of the space. Plantation tourist historian Mary Ann Sternberg, for example, notes that the "name Indian Camp is thought to have double reference: the site once held a Houma village, and the house remained in the Camp family until the latter part of the nineteenth century."[36] When Robert Camp lost the property in 1874, the plantation transitioned into an absentee-owned tenant farm, which remained unused until someone in New Orleans discovered in 1896 the abandoned plantation might become a residence for those removed from the Louisiana Leper Home in the city.[37]

Historian Tiya Miles describes the narratives that emerge from plantation tours, particularly those dedicated to reproducing the plantation as a living archive, as dark tourism.[38] As a contradiction resolved in narrating plantations through slave ghost stories, historic sites that feature, narrate, or memorialize Black ghosts in bondage are ultimately seeking to "engage and yet also avoid the troubling memory of slavery."[39] Such memorialization on former plantation sites, especially those with museums and national status as historic locations like the structures at Carville, allow tourists "to stare and pick at them" while keeping a distance from what they actually represent. They can be witnesses of the story of plantations in the U.S. South without being participants, Miles argues, and therefore be in it without being an actor in the perpetuation of slavery as a "minor story" in the formation of the United States. "Without slavery there is no South, as a region or an idea. Recognition must therefore be a *misrecognition* that diminishes the harsh realities of America's peculiar institution."[40] Marita Sturken describes the acts of witnessing national trauma as an abstraction, as "tourists of history" that mark a distinction from remembering or memory to their actual events, to signify that such tourist subjectivity has "a problematic relationship to the weight, burdens, and meanings of history." Tourism is about "travel that wants to imagine itself as innocent; a tourist is someone who stands outside of a culture, looking at it from a position that demands no responsibility."[41]

As with the other cases discussed in this book, Carville wrestles with the institutional histories of medicine and public health not only in location (broadly defined) but with the contentious memory work in the archive over time. Carville charts a different story about what violence means in such contexts—how it is both remembered and managed through racial logics under national public health. In Carville's specific context, Hansen's disease produced a platform for a national

a

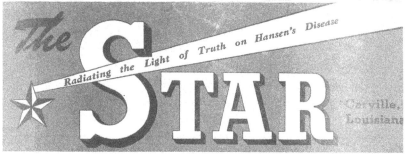

Special Edition Commemorating the 60th Anniversary of this Hospital

Volume 14 No 3   November-December 1954   Price $1.00 per year

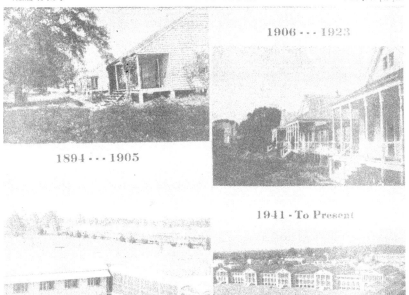

Patients' Quarters Through Sixty Years

FIGURE 4. (a) *Cover of the patient-run newspaper produced at the Carville hospital, the* Star, *vol. 14, no. 3, November–December 1954. The masthead reads "The Star: Radiating the Light of Truth on Hansen's Disease, Carville, Louisiana; Special Edition Commemorating the 60th Anniversary of This Hospital." Below are four photos of the patient quarter over sixty years, the first* (top left) *representing from 1894 to 1905, the second* (top right) *1906–1923, the third* (bottom left) *1924–1940, and the fourth* (bottom right) *1941–Present (1954). The images are aligned with a progress narrative, beginning with a makeshift hospital managed*

Proud Ante-Bellum Mansion Enacts Role In Medical Drama

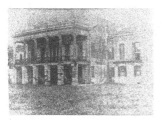

The old plantation mansion built in the year 1854 still stands. Every brick of it was made on the plantation during slave days.

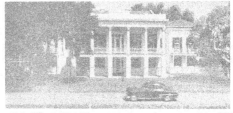

In the 1927 and 1941 building programs, the mansion was renovated and its original design preserved. It serves today as the Administration Building of and administrative, personnel, accounting and finance departments, also office of the Chief Dietician, Director of Nurses, Director of Community Activities; station post office, personnel theatre and an out-patient clinic for hospital personnel. On the first floor are the offices of the Medical Officer in Charge of the hospital.

The second floor houses a medical library, reception room, quarters for single women employees and guest rooms.

Isolated deep in a curve of the Mississippi River at Point Clear* on the levee road about twenty-three miles below Baton Rouge is the old Camp plantation, once one of the proudest sugar plantations on the river, now the site of a U. S. Public Health Service Hospital, the only hospital within continental United States devoted exclusively to the treatment of Hansen's disease.

The old house still stands, minus its many wings and outbuildings, in the center of the great modern institution maintained there now by the government, and serves as a general administration building.

It is painted a glossy white among the dark green of the great live oaks that surround it, and is a superb example of Louisiana architecture with its raised gallery and Corinthian columns upheld by square columns forming a paved portico below, a style found frequently in parts of the state where crevasses were one of the certainties of existence in the middle of the nineteenth century.

The institution occupies the upper part of a tract of land on the lower side of Point Clear. This and adjoining land was assembled into one large estate by Robert C. Camp and known for many years as Indian Camp plantation. The earliest United States land grants confirm the land as having belonged to Walter Burk and Simon Broussard, although it was subject to private ownership for many years previously. In the early days this was known as the St. Gabriel or Manchac section. It was settled by the French, since it was the upper part of the Isle of Orleans claimed by Bienville.

The tract which today holds the peaceful and neatly laid out community was evidently a fertile and productive one, for a study of the title to the place, traced by Will Grace of Plaquemine when the United States Public Health Service bought it in 1921, shows few ownerships and long tenures. The Burk tract went to Jacques Johnson prior to 1809, and Joseph Thomas acquired it from the executors of Johnson's estate on June 26, 1824. It was Johnson who sold it to Camp the following May, and Camp added the Broussard tract to it in 1826 and 1835.

By now Robet Camp, who became General Camp during the War Between the States, had added the entire "Indian Camp" site (so-called because it was once occupied by a part of the Houmas tribe which had its headquarters farther down the river at Burnside) to his estate, which extended 11 arpents or about a mile and a half down the river.

It was Camp who built the mansion there—a glorious structure of some 30 bedrooms, furnished richly throughout with imported furniture, and so beautiful in its stateliness and solitude, beneath its great spreading moss-hung live oaks, that it is still a legend of elegance in that section of the state despite its remoteness and its position off the river road to New Orleans where travelers never pass except by design.

For seventeen years after the mansion was built the Camp family resided at the plantation, which they called Woodlawn and which was so named on Persac's map of the country between New Orleans and Baton Rouge in 1858. Although they lost it later through the financial reverses which came with the downfall of the plantation system, the Camps held the place through the War

Between the States and Reconstruction, living in a style which is still a synonym for luxury and elegance among the descendants of their neighbors on Point Clear.

The Camp family were people of culture and refinement such as only the Old South produced, and they entertained in courtly style, their guests coming by steamboat up the river from New Orleans or overland by horse and carriage, bringing their families and their servants, often remaining for weeks or months at a time. It is still recalled how the people from the plantations around would gather on the levee to watch the carriages go by, bringing the neighborhood gentry when the Camps had one of their receptions.

A sheriff's sale ended the glorious regime of the Camps on April 5, 1874. Henry J. Buddington of New Orleans bid in the place, and his heirs came into possession of the property. At one time during this period it was leased to Douglas Leche of New Orleans, who operated a rice farm there. Ten years later, in March 1884, it was sold to Alphonse Boudeau, who declared its title two years later in favor of Miss Mary Deed Buddington, Miss Kate Charlotte Buddington, and Miss Alice Anne Buddington.

Misses Kate Charlotte and Alice Anne Buddington and the heirs of Miss Mary Deed Buddington, who resided in Paris and never used the plantation, sold the part of the estate where the house stands to the state board of control created to establish a state home for those afflicted with the disease.

Albert G. Phelps was president of this board and acted for it. However,

(Continued on page 22)

from an abandoned slave quarters to several wards accommodating hundreds of patients, doctors, staff, and scientists. (b) An image of an article in the Star, *vol. 14, no. 3, November–December 1954. The article includes two images of the plantation mansion, which was built in 1854, discussing slave plantation history through the narrative of the "War between the States." Box and File no. NHDM 19371.11. Courtesy of National Hansen's Disease Museum, Carville, Louisiana, Permanent Collection.*

conversation about who constitutes the United States citizenry in the twentieth century. This becomes a response to both coloniality and racialized disease, as well as to the global constitution of race converging in medical discourse. Furthermore, Priscilla Wald notes that communicable diseases "know no borders," meaning that investments in nation-states and their economies are challenged by contagion narratives to remake global relations in terms of the "biological scale on which all people and populations are connected."[42] To help explain why the nation serves as the dominant platform for communal formation, Wald turns to Benedict Anderson's theorization of imagined communities to argue that germ theory finds similar traction in the form of national imaginaries, or imagined immunities, as an operative lens: "While emerging infections are inextricable from global interdependence in all versions of these accounts, however, the threat they pose requires a national response. The community to be protected is thereby configured in cultural and political as well as biological terms: the nation as immunological ecosystem. The logic of those terms runs much deeper than state mechanisms and inflects the conception of community articulated in the narratives. Outbreak narratives actually make the act of imagining the community a central (rather than obscured) feature of its preservation."[43] Official documents and records, such as the congressional hearings discussed at the beginning of this chapter, provide one sense of sociality that clarifies national discourse in relation to place, space, policy, and law. Yet, those narratives might also be read against themselves to press on other repositories of memory and representation, such as the problem of critical memory in cultural texts like memoir and essays making meaning of those experiences. What occurs when those histories are narrated through patient memory, particularly as a racialized experience?

Carville and the Problem of Patient Memory

Memoirs by patients at Carville became a popularized phenomenon, with Betty Martin's 1950 *Miracle at Carville: The Story of One Girl's Triumph over the Most Feared Malady* and Stanley Stein's 1963 *Alone No Longer: The Story of a Man Who Refused to Be One of the Living Dead!* serving as templates of sorts for patient activism in that space. In the Stanley Stein papers held at the museum, deeper tensions are at work.

The archive holds the record of residents' lives in the mid-twentieth century, while marking multiple contradictions around race and criminality. In addition to Stein and the archive he curated over years, two others living at Carville as resident patients are covered in the remainder of this chapter: José P. Ramirez Jr. and Josefina "Joey" Guerrero. Ramirez's 2009 memoir *Squint: My Journey with Leprosy,* much like Stein's memoir, is its own kind of archive, and I treat both as such. Josefina "Joey" Guerrero, however, did not write about her own experience in memoir form; she worked over the years for the resident-run newspaper the *Star,* while residing on the grounds, archiving, and often writing about other patients' experiences. Before arriving at Carville, she was the center of a highly publicized case in the United States. Guerrero in fact became known as the wartime patriot heroine in the Philippines who, in the 1940s, as a Filipino resistance fighter, used visual manifestations of Hansen's disease on her body to avoid physical inspection by occupying Japanese soldiers in Manila. This allowed her to smuggle maps and other intelligence to U.S. soldiers, an act that prompted journalists, military writers, and religious (Catholic) advocates to refer to her condition as "Joey's unfortunate passport." Ironically, while this was a reference to the transgressive borders of occupied Manila, it also became the basis on which Guerrero's U.S. citizenship would be obtained in order to be treated at the Carville Leprosarium. This could not have happened without medical and national narratives coming together, as the immigration restrictions put in place by the Johnson-Reed Immigration Act of 1924 made entering the United States via the Philippines nearly impossible.

In Stein's memory of the 1930s and 1940s, whiteness becomes an explicit currency for medical citizenship. Describing his participation in Blackface theater at Carville, he remembers this act of racial mimicry as his attempt to "re-experience the exact point" at which he "decided to begin a campaign to rejoin the human race"—a project that describes how he might become "a naturalized citizen of Carville."[44] Given his own description of losing "anonymity" and "humanity" through the institutionalization process, the performances interrogate the racial dynamics of using Blackface to regain a notion of naturalized citizenship, a notion of belonging that is dependent on making certain claims to whiteness. Recent histories have held that the Carville Leprosarium produced a space that resisted the social and political realities of white supremacy of the time. Referring to Carville as "an ethnic melting pot," Claire Manes notes that the hospital accepted international patients: "men, women, and children from not only the United States but from locations as diverse as Japan, Puerto Rico, Mexico, and the Philippines." Manes goes as far as to suggest that the "ethnic mix were united by the microbes that had invaded their bodies."[45] Stein's account of Carville, however, suggests formations that relied heavily on the notion that whiteness was an explicit form of property.

STANLEY STEIN

Sidney Maurice Levyson (alias Stanley Stein), born in Gonzalez, Texas, charts his transformation from what he describes as a relatively ordinary life in a secular Jewish family to a Hansen's disease patient and patient rights activist. This transformation began the first day he entered the hospital. Upon his arrival, the Sisters of Charity asked for his new name for hospital records, a routine practice implemented to protect patients' family members from stigmatization. Stein remembers walking through his thoughts: "Another name? What was wrong with my own name? Did I have to hide under an alias like a hunted criminal?"[46] In response to his newly assigned number, he claims he "would always be No. 746, a number identified not only with my case history but with everything I would do at Carville for the next third of the century. . . . I was sinking into the quagmire of anonymity which society reserves for the victims of leprosy, mental illness, or crime. We were no more entitled to individuality than a convict in a penitentiary."[47] Typical in memoirs of disease, contagion, and quarantine, the discursive power to transform autonomous bodies into prisoner-patients is a central component. The shift from name to number, from a person with unquestioned value to a devalued medical subject, from "individuality" to "anonymity," are what Stein highlights as constructed, naturalized categories only acceptable for those labeled "diseased," "disabled," and "criminal."

Sidonie Smith and Julia Watson suggest that such "narrative acts of reclaiming" a medically stigmatized or objectified body often resist situating the body as abnormative, ultimately serving as a "critique of the damaged body as a social construction of Western medicine."[48] More recently, James Kyung-Jin Lee's reflection on Asian American illness memoir describes this particular genre of life writing as serving as the writing act that allows for the writer to rediscover a particular notion of selfhood in the context of medicalization. While Lee's focus is on contemporary Asian American memoir and its relationship to neoliberal logics, the question of what illness memoir makes possible is useful for this discussion. Lee writes:

> Memoirs, as idiosyncratic as the people who write them, are narrative actions of "participation in the public sphere." . . . So, like their authors, memoirs are fragile objects, easily misunderstood or dismissed for presumed lower quality or unexamined bias or grandeurs of celebrity. But even with the rise of so many platforms for communication and communicability, such as blogs, social media, and personal websites, there is an inverse relation to the valuation of selfhood. Asian Americans strive to find themselves in U.S. society, and their constricted form of recognition is a model minority suit, off-the-rack or bespoke. People get sick and go to the doctor and are ordered to take off their clothes and slip into a gown whose openness feels universally invasive; they soon learn that they are little more than a litany of symptoms and prognoses, at risk of losing their narrative anchor and temporality.[49]

Where Lee locates memoir as a potentiality for relating differently with the self—that is, beyond the market-driven world of memoir that we know today, which necessarily imagines real-time audiences—he also sees the genre of memoir providing, in the act of writing, those who have "experienced the profanities of existential loss, the work of re-enchantment of the 'I' in the self and of sharing this reimagined 'I' with another."[50] Because the genre itself presumes access to interiority, whether in the form of confessionals, revealing vulnerabilities, or journeys through transformations, Lee is most interested in exploring the dimensions beyond what he calls medical ontologies—the process of medicalization that generally seeks to replace the "life" of a person with the figure of a medical patient, as Lee puts it, "even as, phenomenologically, such 'life' appears less and less human."[51] Instead, he suggests that memoirs insist on being read and heard differently, not only as self-discoveries but as acts of commitment to self and others.[52]

The connections in Stein's memoir between being denied "individuality" and the mundane activities that make up institutional life, "seeking laxative tablets and making a laundry list," solidify for Stein the transformative power of this space as it works to make "criminals" behind bars (i.e., nonpersons) out of sick people. In other words, making public the production of prisoner-patients in the context of Hansen's disease requires inhabiting the role, examining the reimagined "I" that the memoir produces, and then speaking from within it. Yet, what happens when we ask how this new self emerges, under what conditions it is made possible, particularly with relation to race and racialization? Stein's passages above represent the scenes of prisoner-patient life; it is the moments of transformation throughout the memoir that deserve a bit more examination. The most explicit moment of what Stein describes as regaining his humanity provides telling examples of how disease is racialized, even through memory.

Provocatively using the Little Theater—an amateur patient troupe at Carville intended to entertain the doctors, nurses, staff, and other patients—as the platform to narrativize the performance of self, Stein describes a theater role in Blackface as a site of transformation. It was the "success of the minstrel show [that] made me a naturalized citizen of Carville. The smell of grease paint had done me more good than Fowler's Solution. The rehearsals had led to two-way friendships. . . . Strangers stopped me on the boardwalks to say hello. Doctors and nurses smiled at me as we passed."[53]

Some explore that such moments signal a reconfiguration of race, belonging, currency, and property produced by constructing whiteness against Blackness through Blackface performance in medical spaces. In *Theaters of Madness: Insane Asylums and Nineteenth-Century American Culture,* for example, Benjamin Reiss suggests that Blackface performance in nineteenth-century asylums enabled white men, who were diagnosed as "insane," to lay claim to their capacity of "self-control." In a patient performance at the New York State Lunatic Asylum, performed during the 1840s and 1850s, Reiss notes that white patients "enacted scenarios of slave life for the ultimate captive audience; and under the watchful eye of the asylum authorities, they turned a famously unruly form into a spectacle of their own capacity for self-control. From behind Blackface masks, they spoke to each other, to their doctors (who doubled as their captors), to the curious townsfolk and even politicians who were occasionally given admittance [to minstrel performances]."[54] Michael Rogin situates Blackface performance of the nineteenth and twentieth centuries as offering a disavowal between Jewish ethnic identity and Blackness, opportunities to leverage a familiar narrative of turning failure into success, turning punishment into new forms of economic, social, racial, and cultural capital. Alternative racial roots "are not arbitrary, for just as the frontier period in American history generated the classic American literature, so American film was born in the industrial age out of the conjunction between southern defeat in the Civil War, black resubordination, and national integration; the rise of the multiethnic, industrial metropolis; and the emergence of mass entertainment, expropriated from its black roots, as the locus of Americanization."[55] Rogin traces just such racial transformation, examining the "conjunction between blackface and Americanization" as the enabling factor in entering American conceptions of whiteness. Indeed, Saidiya Hartman's important examination of white abolitionist capacity to imagine humanity as depending on imagining, and inhabiting in writing, Black suffering interrogates the benevolent narration of humanitarian questions about Blackness being interpreted under the category of "human." Hartman explores the thought of white presbyterian minister and abolitionist John Rankin, whose writings imagined the suffering of enslaved people: "Rankin becomes a proxy and the other's pain is acknowledged to the degree that it can be imagined, yet by virtue of this substitution the object of identification threatens to disappear. In order to convince the reader of the horrors of slavery, Rankin must volunteer himself and his family for abasement. Put differently, the effort to counteract the commonplace callousness to black suffering requires that the white body be positioned in the place of the black body in order to make this suffering visible and intelligible."[56]

Stein's work as a Carville disability rights activist in the space extends far beyond that particular geography, as he dedicates his life to dismantling several long-standing policies, discourses, and narratives that have dehumanized and stigmatized nonnormative bodies. Indeed, the Stanley Stein Archive at the National Hansen's Disease Museum is the focus of many who have sought to narrate the importance of the political work that happened there. That archive, created by Stein and managed by those who understand its importance, has yet to be analyzed and considered in ways that it deserves to be. Those future examinations, however, ought to hold in tension the many contradictions

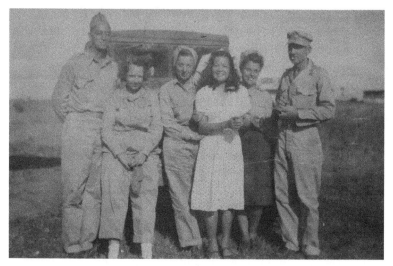

FIGURE 5. *Joey Guerrero poses in front of a military jeep with U.S. Army nurses. Details unknown. Courtesy of National Hansen's Disease Museum, Carville, Louisiana, Permanent Collection.*

within it, looking to texts and traces left by figures such as Guerrero and Ramirez.

JOSEFINA "JOEY" GUERRERO

Josefina "Joey" Guerrero, a friend of the *Star*'s editor, Stanley Stein, points to other performances. A member of the underground resistance movement during Japanese occupation of Manila, Guerrero became famous in the United States for using her "unfortunate passport"—referring to the visible manifestations of Hansen's disease on her face and body. This bodily passport provided her access into Japanese-occupied territories in order to deliver U.S. soldiers maps and other strategic intelligence. Guerrero was widely praised for smuggling hidden maps and documents through checkpoints and other guarded areas to warn U.S. troops of recently mined areas.

In 1949, George Doody published a letter in the *Wanderer* to convince U.S. readers of Guerrero's patriotism and heroism:

> By the muddy waters of Old Man River, about sixty miles north of
> New Orleans, you will find the little town of Carville, La., and the

U.S. Marine Hospital—our National Leprosarium—operated by the U.S. Public Health Service. A guest there is one of the truly great and inspiring personalities of our time—little Joey Guerrero, the darling leper heroine of the Philippine campaign, who, through her heroism in the war with Japan, saved thousands of American lives. For her services to our Armed Forces she has been awarded the highest civilian decoration of the U.S. Government—the Medal of Freedom with Silver Palm. On orders of the Attorney General Tom Clark, she was transferred from the pathetic leper colony at Novaliches, near Manila, P.I., to Carville, La., where modern facilities are available.... To honor this "Joan of Arc" of the Pacific War and to provide the means to make it possible for her to carry on her corporal works of mercy for lepers—on an international scale—"Joey's International Leprosy Fund" was organized. We appeal to "Joey's" buddies of the 37th Division—and all others who appreciate what this little leper heroine did to save our skins during the late war—to write to us and help promote the cause of leprosy, which "Joey" personifies.[57]

The United States officially recognized Guerrero with its highest civilian medal, which gained her admittance to the Carville hospital as "the first foreign patient" to be treated there. For over a decade, Guerrero's case and her "right to U.S. citizenship" were discussed and debated in newspapers and on television, in congressional bills, featured in *Time* magazine, as well as in the war histories and accounts into the 1960s. Guerrero's welcome was bolstered by ongoing World War II gendered narratives of white saviors, such as Thomas Johnson's 1963 essay "Joey's Quiet War." After years of appeals from military officers, priests, politicians, and Filipino patients at Carville, her transfer was approved with "a heroine's welcome" on July 11, 1948.[58] Guerrero's arrival attracted news media and government public relations attention, and while much of those archives are lost, some remnants have surfaced over the years, including footage recorded at her U.S. arrival (Figure 6).

Stein describes Guerrero's situation as gaining access to certain privileges, all of which were threatened by deportation:

[She] wanted an American diploma. In fact, she wanted to become an American citizen. Having been admitted to the U.S. under an exception to the immigration laws, she realized that her status was

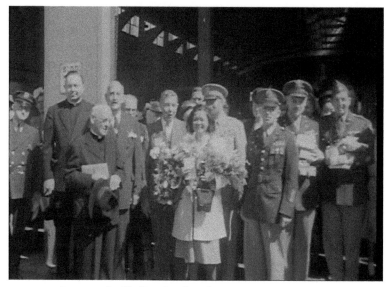

FIGURE 6. *A newsreel still of Josefina "Joey" Guerrero arriving in the United States in 1948. "Mrs Guerrero—Heroine of Filipino Underground," Film ID 2457.24, Reuters via British Pathé.*

precarious and that she might face deportation proceedings at the whim of a bureaucrat in a new administration. *The Star* and our American Legion friends went to bat for the girl who had risked death to save hundreds of American lives in the Philippines. Congressman James Morrison introduced a bill into the House (HR 2960) which would have given Joey U.S. citizenship, but memories of the war in the Pacific were getting a little dim on Capitol Hill and heroism was its own reward anyhow. HR 2960 died in Committee.[59]

Memories of the Pacific, in all accounts of this event, structured the notion of citizenship that became central to narrating Guerrero's value within the U.S. wartime context. At Carville, Guerrero became a patient advocate working with the *Star* and pursued education to remove herself from the spotlight. When Guerrero enrolled in a correspondence course offered by a fashion academy, Stein notes she "got her check back with a note saying: 'Because of your wonderful service to your own government as well as that of the United States, we are extending you a scholarship in the Home Study Division.'"[60] The public figure of Joey circulated widely, and she eventually changed her name and moved to California to gain some control over her life.

JOSÉ P. RAMIREZ JR.

José P. Ramirez Jr.'s *Squint: My Journey with Leprosy,* while written more recently and published in 2009, connects the longer historical memory of Carville to questions surrounding slavery, dispossession, and Jim Crow. Unlike other Carville memoirs, Ramirez insists that those histories continue to live on to haunt the present. Attempting to make sense of the stigmas of disease as they converge with various forms of racism and segregation, Ramirez observes that the hospital grounds at Carville were "divided into two worlds," one for the diseased and one for the nondiseased.[61] "This area [of the facility], which had over twenty buildings, mostly cottages for public health service staff and visitors, was off limits to us residents of the 'other' world." Ramirez's "two worlds" is quickly linked to Jim Crow: "I was able to meet only a few of the children who lived on the station, but I always wondered what their thoughts were about growing up in Louisiana where segregation by race was a common practice, and then residing on the hospital grounds where segregation due to illness was commonly accepted."[62] Ramirez chronicles his early struggles to find medical treatment in the United States, while also dealing with stigmatization surrounding Hansen's disease in Mexico. As a teenager in the 1960s, he traveled to the Carville Leprosarium, recalling the details of his displacement and ostracization by several communities. Ramirez wonders about this space as a site of temporal traversing of spatial imaginaries—"sick" and racialized experiences converging over time in Ramirez's memory. The details that tell the history of Carville serve as backdrop to the story of unjust or undeserving incarceration experiences that have little to do with the racial dynamics of the space. However, Ramirez develops a more nuanced critique of the longer historical memory as it stands in the present. What were the thoughts of children who grew up "where segregation by race was the common practice," and how does this process register an ongoing relationship to white supremacy? When Ramirez reads the "common practice" with "segregation due to illness," it suggests an engagement with narratives not of a distant past but of a haunted present. Indeed, Cheryl Harris argues that such ahistorical fantasies work part and parcel with colorblind ideologies of the contemporary moment, which hold sway in legal and popular discourse, pointing to discussion of "race and racism in the past tense."[63]

Ramirez again grounds the connection by commenting on the tension in framing the history of Carville as a national project, narrated through tourist facts that situated moments as dead and all but forgotten. The official narrative of Carville is, in part, represented by monuments like the plantation mansion, but more so by national plaques and historical narratives on display. A plaque outside of the property, for example, reads: "Indian Camp Plantation: The plantation home, built in the 1850's, became the site of the Louisiana State Leprosarium in 1894. The U.S. Public Health Service acquired it in 1921. It is now known as the National Hansen's Disease Center." Ramirez's memoir often refuses to naturalize the space through memorialization, instead reading against the record: "The oval design [of the Carville buildings], according to the National Register of Historic Places, mimicked the 'footprint that the former slave cabins occupied' on the Indian Camp Plantation."[64] Inscribed into the design of the National Leprosarium is the naming of the living space, but it also names those who inhabited those quarters. Put differently, Ramirez's account circles around the plantation palimpsest.

Conclusion

This chapter asserts that the tension framing Carville is also explicit in cultural production and memory work, as is stated in this passage of Michelle Cliff's *Free Enterprise*: "The official version is in everybody's mouth.... This is what happened; this is how it was."[65] Memory, however, finds traction in the lives of patients who found themselves, at different times and for different reasons, living at the National Leprosarium, and it does so in more complex ways than what the problem of law or public health policy presents to its publics. Considering more closely the function of knowledge production in patient memoir and the archives that capture other forms of memory helps to reconsider what race and criminality offer up in the form of crafted remembering. Memoir, or life narrative, can be understood as a "source, authenticator, and destabilizer of autobiographical acts," where memory negotiates scientific narrative differently, ultimately unsettling it.[66] In the case of Carville, cultural text and memory connect medical knowledge about the transmission of Hansen's disease, as discussed in the previous chapter on other sites and locations, with forms of state-sanctioned violence, settler colonialism, and a particular form of racial capital and possession as it manifests through medicine and public health. While the previous chapter focused on the prisoner-patient as a "valid example of experimental inoculation," this chapter focused on the interplay between the public health institutions in Hawai'i—those that became a part of a larger conversation about the United States—and the role Louisiana Carville National Leprosarium played in the present.[67]

One problem of narrating Carville's public history is that, as an institution, it cannot dwell on the conditions that have made it possible for medicine to thrive and to be triumphant. Rather, to narrate its progress in history is to highlight the scientific work that cured Hansen's disease and the triumph of patients who navigated forced quarantine, public health laws, and so on, and to subsume the materiality of that progress. The narrative is charting the past as the successes of medicine, securing a story that contributes to ideas of a U.S. nation-state. To achieve this, it must not remove the settler-colonial project from the narrative of the United States but naturalize it within a teleological origin story.

CHAPTER 3

Imagining Medical Archives at Olive View

A better term might have been a prison.

—IRWIN ZIMENT, CHIEF OF MEDICINE AT
OLIVE VIEW–UCLA MEDICAL CENTER

The sanatorium is jail. I'm not being treated here. I'm being punished! I'm a political prisoner because I suffer from a political disease!

—ALEJANDRO MORALES, *THE CAPTAIN OF
ALL THESE MEN OF DEATH*

The October 28, 1995, issue of the *Los Angeles Times* covered the seventy-fifth anniversary celebration of the Olive View Sanatorium in Sylmar, California. At the reopening celebration, the *Times* reporter observed: "There were speeches and cake Friday to honor the hospital that has been transformed into a modern facility from a collection of wood-frame buildings where the sick and dying tuberculosis patients were forced by law to stay."[1] With interviews of the former medical staff and surviving patients who attended the event, the article narrates the inauguration of the new medical facilities, which were built to replace the old residential wards and buildings erected in the 1920s, as a celebration. The story quickly turns, however, to the participants' memories of a distinctly violent, carceral experience. The chief of medicine at Olive View, Irwin Ziment, for instance, notes that while the sanatorium was always known as a center of medical innovation, perhaps "a better term [for the sanatorium] might have been a priso[n]."[2] Former patients depicted their postdiagnosis TB experiences as systematic subjection to "horrifying and probably ineffective treatments" and noted their experience was "like being in jail." Others remembered a prisonlike experience in which doctors and Los Angeles County public health officials could have people arrested with "a stroke of the pen." While acknowledging these unsettling policies and practices, director J. P. Myles Black maintained that many officials understood these police actions as necessary to protect the public: "They had to be controlled. Not because they had a disease, but because they were spreading it." Director Black identifies the threat as being found largely with "salad makers, waiters, [and] dishwashers."

During the first half of the twentieth century, Southern California had established firm foundations on which to think about race through the lenses of citizenship, disease, and containment, finding currency in the institution of public health. In 1944, for example, the medical journal *California and Western Medicine* published the short public health essay "Migratory Agricultural Workers of California: Their Health Care," which, along with other medical journals, attempted to draw attention to so-called threats emanating from Mexican and Mexican American communities working in and around Los Angeles.[3] At a moment of heightened suburbanization across the United States, where suburbs grew exponentially faster than city centers, the article voices the urgent concern for the medical community to respond to the ways California's agricultural industry affected its city dwellers, emphasizing the Los Angeles area as an important site of concern.[4] It does this by bringing together exaggerated stories that circulated around poor, racialized laborers, substandard living conditions at migrant labor camps, contagious diseases, and the nation's duty to protect the state. The article cautions readers:

> Physicians need not stretch their imagination to visualize how such itinerant [Mexican] workers, who are often poorly nourished and diseased, when grouped together under conditions not by any means sanitary, may become a menace not only to themselves, but so to the citizens of nearby communities, and so to the people of the State at large.[5]

The article frames this as protecting the public, yet the scenario depicted depends on physicians holding back the impulse to imagine a threat ("need not stretch their imagination") so they may see ("visualize") the actual threat that exists before them. The statement cautions those positioned to protect the state from this immanently real danger, while at the same time it imagines, indeed, conjures up, an enemy of the state—one that traveled from south of the U.S.–Mexico borderlands, is positioned to infect "citizens of nearby communities," and therefore urgently needs containing.

Public health agents perceived such scenarios as threats not only to residents of Los Angeles but also to people living in other large cities across the state. There was, the *California and Western Medicine* article suggests, an urgent need to deal with the "thousands of needy agricultural workers, both those who are residents of California and the larger number who voluntarily, or through Federal aid as in the case of the Mexicans, are brought into the State."[6] While physicians and scientists debated how migrant labor shifted policy focus around race and disease, contributors to medical journals of the time often entangled and conflated public health and public security as social goods and necessary evils. In the 1940s, *California and Western Medicine* was one of several influential medical and scientific journals presenting authoritative notions that the "thousands of needy [Mexican] agricultural workers"— Mexican workers in California before and after the establishment of the Bracero Program (1942–1965)—could be dealt with as a single homogeneous group, "poorly nourished and diseased," and "a menace not only to themselves" but potentially to the whole of the United States. The article was taking part in an ongoing debate in medicine and public health over this "menace," often referred to as "the Mexican problem."[7] Such print culture helped to produce and grant legitimacy to ideas about how the built environment emerged in response to perceived threats as spaces of protection and as technologies of containment.

This chapter examines the production of racialized disease in a California public health context by placing it in dialogue with the memories of patients depicted in Chicanx fiction. Alejandro Morales's 2008 novel *The Captain of All These Men of Death* centers collective memories of the Los Angeles Olive View Sanatorium in the 1940s and 1950s as a contested space of uneasy belonging. Building on scholarship in critical medical studies and cultural studies, I look to Morales's novel because it presents a platform for interpreting patient experiences documenting the logics of medicine from a cultural point of view. By doing so, the novel unsettles narratives produced within official accounts of U.S. medical science. *The Captain* recasts those racial, political, and social categories that undergird the policies of public health and security to instead foreground the lived experiences of communities affected most by those medical institutions. The novel, in other words, makes those narratives central to the production of their own histories, while at the same time it interprets acts of medical violence as constitutive to narratives of scientific progress and benevolence. The novel explores the temporalities of medical technologies, the lives that live within them, and the ways racialized patients were both moved through and contained in what I am calling carceral health imaginaries. Arguing for a more robust understanding of what constitutes the medical archive, this chapter suggests that the past remains deeply contested at the intersections of culture and exists where cultural production remembers against the firm, often immovable scientific record. Within the larger framework of *Archiving Medical Violence,* one goal of this chapter is to put some pressure on the structures of hierarchized knowledge, to interrogate its stabilizing effect on the archive, and to reconsider things not often understood as part of the official record.

Race and Disease in Los Angeles

The compounded impact of racialized disease, as a discourse that marks a threat to white Californians, animates public health to shift more directly to bolster white settler protections. Those official shifts were understood largely as acts to secure the public through law, carried out by respected and powerful figures in medicine.[8] Natalia Molina traces connections between medical diagnosis and policing, detaining, and deporting migrant labor in California. Molina maps the ways in which policing technologies were refined to "mark undesirable immigrant groups as outsiders."[9] Alexandra Minna Stern highlights those regularized exclusionary practices targeting racialized communities, suggesting that they were not at all fringe acts carried out by "hacks and mad scientists."[10] Indeed, Ruha Benjamin shows that those acts were consistently orchestrated by "prominent doctors, philanthropists, journalists, academicians, and administrators who wished to amplify the reach of an extensive eugenics agenda that dated back to the turn of the century."[11] As discussed in previous chapters, what produced notions that medicine could self-govern and transgress laws with impunity came from, in part, the ability to carry on robust dialogues while operating in relative isolation and away from the scrutiny of a broader public.[12] Unearthing and rereading municipal archives, specifically those that saw public health as an issue of state or national security, brings such exclusionary mechanisms into sharper view.

In the early twentieth century, Los Angeles intensified efforts to target and criminalize entire groups of Mexican and Mexican American workers and communities around the understanding that communicable diseases needed to be contained. Sociological research played a significant role in developing these ideas, as historian David Gutiérrez notes. In 1928, the Los Angeles County Health Department developed a housing stock numerical rating system for the county, finding Mexicans' residential patterns to be "the worst in the area."[13] Rates of infection by communicable disease—tuberculosis, in particular—were intimately tied to living conditions and the city's efforts to exclude. Similarly, Vicki Ruiz asserts that labor and living conditions for racialized communities in Los Angeles have often been tied to narratives surrounding contagious disease. Ruiz points to sanitation policies to clarify this point, noting that the work of "social scientists, Protestant missionaries, and social workers uniformly deplore the overcrowded, unsanitary conditions in which Mexicans were compelled to live."[14] Molina argues that the conflation of racial identity and contagious disease, specifically in relation to Chinese, Japanese, and Mexican communities in the late nineteenth and early twentieth centuries, began in the 1870s, prompting a steady pattern among city health officials that connected "any blemish on the pristine image of Los Angeles—including all forms of disease and any manner of disorder—to the city's marginalized communities."[15] Scientific authority was more firmly anchored in the institutionalization of public health as a securitizing imperative, tasked with protecting the city from communicable disease. Molina shows how this task was woven into the shored-up xenophobic duty of removing "rotten spots" (i.e., ethnic communities) from a raced and gendered public.

The archival trace of racialized exclusion in Los Angeles government records rested firmly on the backs of Mexican communities, and the county Department of Health aggressively sought out reasons to narrate high rates of tuberculosis in those communities specifically as a racialized discourse. To that end, statistical documentation overwhelmed the discussion, selectively framing Mexican Americans as the city's public health threat, burden, and obstacle to investment in public resources. Emily K. Abel observes that public health records indicate that government funding for tuberculosis care nearly vanished during the Depression. The resource-burden narrative that blamed excessive health care for Mexicans in Olive View, as well as in city and county clinics, prompted nativist politicians and policymakers to argue against allocating funds for poor residents.[16] Through public health campaigns, this notion played a crucial role in creating the figure of representative disease-carrying Mexicans in the form of brown bodies. Molina points to one such example, where public health and the protection of the public were usefully confused—what she describes as the moment when public health as a science is blurred as a public service, demonstrating how the language of scientific research could and does "bleed into policy considerations."[17] Overseeing the operations of Olive View, the Department of Charities conducted a study that resulted in a report featuring a Mexican immigrant couple with tuberculosis. The report alleged that the couple infected eighty-three people, all reported to be members of the couple's own family network. Such depictions positioned Mexicans as a burden to the public health system and a racialized contagious threat to a so-called general public. These imaginaries extended nativist, eugenicist conceptions of race in the mainstream, leading to more aggressive uses of public health as a tool of quarantine, deportation, and incarceration.[18]

Prior to the 1924 Immigration Act (discussed in chapter 2), which placed restrictions on so-called undesirable groups migrating to the United States, there were significantly fewer concerns about stopping movement into the United States from Mexico. The decades following this legislation mark an important shift in the perception of Mexican laborers from "a racially inferior but generally malleable workforce" to the intensified and enduring representations of Mexicans as "criminal, a social burden, diseased, and inassimilable."[19] Furthermore, Mexican laborers were regularly identified as foreign, despite their status as residents, laborers, or citizens. In some cases, families were quarantined and subjected to experimental treatments, including those influenced by collapsed lung theory, which induced the collapse of the lung by surgically removing rib bones.[20] While tuberculosis was often discussed in public health educational programs as an indiscriminate killer—infecting equally across social, racial, and cultural categories—the conflation of tuberculosis with race, class, gender, and nationality sig-

nificantly shaped policy and practice. Public health in the early twentieth century advances yet another carceral technology in Los Angeles,
where race and citizenship provided useful and effective frameworks
for policing and containing racialized populations. Indeed, this carceral imaginary narrates the necessity of containing, quarantining,
removing, and cutting out what is perceived as the rot of public space.

Reframing the official scientific record, these histories help not only
to confront a dominant perception of the role of medicine—that it is, at
its core, a benevolent and humanitarian endeavor—but also to critically
examine the outcomes of archival knowledge, the definitions of progress in use, and the visions of futurity contained within. Reconsidering
archival knowledge in this way—what it is, who it belongs to, and where
it is sanctioned—sheds light on racial, ableist, gendered, and settler-
colonial logics maintaining it. In this context, I look to Alejandro
Morales's novel *The Captain of All These Men of Death* as a cultural text
that reconfigures narratives of progress and individual freedom to consider what resistance in the archive can reveal, and to do so without
seeking to resolve archival contradictions.[21] The "terrain of the national
culture," Lisa Lowe argues, functions as a site of immersion into "the
repertoire of American memories, events, and narratives," simultaneously locating the terrain where hierarchical dynamics of social, legal,
and political representation in the United States are worked out and in
the space for collective memory to negotiate otherwise.[22] While law is
perhaps the one that most literally governs citizenship through "collec-
tively forged images, histories, and narratives that place, displace, and
replace individuals in relation to the national polity," cultural production has the potential to rewrite those scripts and to shape how people
forget and remember. To center more expansive forms of resistance
around refusal and remembering across antiracist, feminist, and migrant experiences presents questions differently, allowing an inquiry
through unlikely temporalities, memories, and cultural representation.

Critical Memory and *The Captain of All These Men of Death*

The Captain of All These Men of Death begins in the 1990s with the protagonist, Robert Contreras, casually addressing readers with reflections
about his life: "You see, nothing really exciting happened in my life. I led
a normal life. The strangest thing that happened was when my nephew

came to visit with his son, who asked me for an interview."[23] The interview, conducted by the author and his son, Gregory Morales, sought to record his experiences at Olive View Sanatorium (now the Olive View–UCLA Medical Center) from the mid-1940s to the mid-1950s as research for Gregory's medical thesis and cultural history of tuberculosis. In part, the novel was inspired by the actual UCLA med-school thesis written by Gregory Morales.[24] Both the thesis and Alejandro Morales's novel engage the history of Olive View Sanatorium, the people who lived and worked there, and the cultural and medical histories that shaped and emerged from the hospital. Robert Contreras, who, as noted in the novel's preface, was modeled after the author's uncle, pieces together buried memories, temporal landscapes, historical pasts and presents—all of which collide as uncollected experiences to make up the novel's fragmented archive of a forgotten moment in Los Angeles history.[25] When thinking back, Contreras recalls the "wonderful images of the past, [like] photos in my mind," evoking depictions of Olive View that resemble photos and illustrated postcards sold to resident patients and their families in the first half of the twentieth century. Those images present the grounds as utopian landscapes, a no-place in the foothills of the Sierra Madre, set outside the Los Angeles city-space and away from the businesses and the general hospital in downtown. The serene pastoral landscapes, like much of Southern California's histories, are designed to remind residents of a romantic eighteenth-century Spanish missionary past, while at the same time very carefully erasing the Indigenous presence and dispossession that the San Fernando Mission manufactured.[26]

From this emerge several tensions between Contreras's recovered experiences as a racialized, wartime tuberculosis patient (a "TBer") and the titanic weight of medical knowledge and authority. The novel shifts to a first-person account, beginning with Contreras's nearly forgotten attempts to enlist in the U.S. Army in 1944. Before he can enlist, the army physician diagnoses Contreras with tuberculosis, which launches him into years of medical surveillance under the Los Angeles Department of Public Health. He is moved from one hospital to another, until finally landing at the Olive View Sanatorium in Sylmar, which was known in the mid-twentieth century as the Los Angeles medical center serving poor, itinerant patients, and it was known nationally as the premier hospital researching the treatment and containment of tuberculosis on the U.S. West Coast. While living as an Olive View patient for nearly a decade, Contreras experiences the mundane routines of patient life, but he also witnesses forced incarceration of suspected TBers, experimental, often fatal medical procedures carried out on poor people of color, and various forms of patient activism and resistance. Through the lens of memory, then, *The Captain* blurs the lines of archival recovery and official documentation of medical violence. Unsettling medical history as the major achievements of scientists and physicians, the novel instead situates settler-colonial histories of the region as the conditions for California medicine, centering individual and collective experiences of racialized patients to tell the story of Olive View.

Scholars discuss Morales's use of historical framing to ground the fictional content as something more than storytelling, and Morales himself has done much in his own writing to undermine the notion that "history" and "fiction" are easily separated.[27] He describes the problem of his work as "an attempt to conjure a fantasy of accuracy inhabited by those persons living or dead who intentionally, by their own free will, with pleasure or torment, read and identify themselves in the story."[28] While at Olive View, for example, Contreras joins the volunteer staff of patient-journalists and contributes to the hospital newspaper *Olive View-Point* as both writer and journalist. Based on the historical publication produced at Olive View Sanatorium, this fictional version of the newspaper traces the history of tuberculosis and its treatment over centuries, showing how the disease affected governments and marginalized communities of both the past and present. Contreras notes that his first writing assignment was to research the Mission San Fernando Valley, significant as a site of settler-colonial histories affecting both disease and the carceral legacies of the Spanish empire.[29] Covered in a story from the actual 1945 issue of *Olive View-Point*, discussed in Gregory Morales's thesis, the attention to this longer arc of history foregrounds the novel's focus on the ways the Los Angeles infrastructure has been built on Tongva territory through settler-colonial logics.[30]

The novel poses several sets of problems for readers to work out: Is medical violence a fact of the past and, if so, of whose past? Is it contained by history, or do those histories haunt the present and continue to structure the future? Perhaps more importantly, what might it mean for a novel so invested in the official histories of the region to take seriously the constitutive relationships between memory and those carceral structures shaping medicine? Characters in this novel, for instance, struggle to come to terms with their own fidelities to medical authority and, at the same time, to confront the reality that racialized bodies have long histories of being used as raw materials for scientific experimentation and advancement. As Stuart Hall suggests, when imagining the ways to "break, contest or interrupt some of these tendential historical connections, you have to know when you are moving against the grain of historical formations." Likewise, moving or rearticulating those narratives means drawing the needle across "all the grooves that have articulated [them] already."[31] The novel questions the definitions of progress underpinning the narration of science and medicine as a humanistic project, but it does so by rearticulating it as a racial project. Contreras suggests, in other words, that the power of historical scripts animating medical science as a benevolent force helps to explain, in part, how race and class intersect to create the conditions for medical violence: "Frankly, knowing the histories of these buildings sheds a completely different perspective on what having tuberculosis was and meant, on what medicine was and has accomplished, on how medicine became abusive and how the patients, especially those of us who were poor, Mexican, and black kept our mouths shut and didn't say a word about what the doctors and nurses did to us. Unfortunately, all this was so easily forgotten."[32]

Describing "another side of the tuberculosis crusade," Contreras suggests that "the willingness of tuberculants to be test patients, sanatorium guinea pigs, or experimental rats" has everything to do with how they are racialized and specifically how that process situates entire groups as powerless within the larger structures of medicine.[33] Contreras continues:

A dangerous selfishness compelled them to try any experimental drug presented to them. "If it works, I'll be the first to be cured!" I overheard their justifications, their rationalization as they swallowed, injected, inhaled, or worse, went up to La Loma for experimental surgery. Aware of the possibility of disastrous setbacks such as devastating physical abnormalities or fatal unexpected reactions, they became desperate and eagerly accepted whatever the doctors suggested. They were no longer willing or capable of struggling with the drudgery of their illness, and being bedridden had become overwhelmingly intolerable. . . . I could see it in their faces, in their calm demeanor: they were happy about their decision to be cured or die as quickly as possible.[34]

Olive View patients willing to consent to experimental drugs has connections with Gregory Morales's medical thesis: "Olive View itself was a testing ground for all these drugs and it is clear from the monthly newsletter that the patients waited anxiously for their chance to try the drugs."[35] Throughout the medical thesis, Morales turns to several *Olive View-Point* issues as an alternative to more conventional (empirical) medical reports. He finds, for example, one documentation of patient desire to participate in drug experimentation in "The Munson Lament"—a poem written by a patient and published in the *Olive View-Point.* Perhaps obviously significant in that these narratives were likely not commonly recorded elsewhere, the impulse, as a student of medicine, to read the archive through patient expression might be read as making possible the future novel by his father and its critical interrogations of scientific archival knowledge.

In Alejandro Morales's novel *The Captain,* the possibility of consenting to such experimental medicines becomes more fraught as patients existing on the margins are either disappeared or killed, nearly always with impunity.[36] Contreras notices that patients, overnight, "would be gone with no explanation," and that "being queer was a risky, dangerous business." The social realities demonstrate yet another layer of medical violence, where one could be "isolated, ignored, denied treatment, be found dead suddenly and mysteriously, or [be] murdered."[37] The novel works to detail the ways in which patients, particularly those who were most vulnerable to death or disappearance, emerged from and contributed to medical violence. Contreras continues to critically observe the lives of Mexican, Black, women, and queer patients, as well as patients with "a reputation of being a subversive, a political or social troublemaker on the outside."[38] Such patients would go up to La Loma—the surgical unit and large laboratory that blocked the view of the experimental ward, a place that "reminded everyone of Frankenstein and his castle where the good doctor had created a monster"—never to be seen again. "What I didn't know," Contreras confesses as he remembers this time of his life, "was that they weren't always taken up there only for surgery, but also for tests, chemical experiments."[39]

The novel itself, then, emerges as a catalog of medical misery and carceral memory, listing not only Contreras's observations but those of many patients over several years. Narrating his first encounter with La Loma, Contreras recalls meeting with Consuelo Anzur, a patient who "had signed a waiver to participate in testing a new drug." Another patient and friend of Consuelo explains, "She didn't know what she was doing. They scared her and got her to do it. She barely understands English. She has no relatives, no friends, nobody to check on her. The experimental drug made her worse." Finally, urging Contreras to leverage the newspaper as a political tool, she says: "Put this in the *Point*, Bob. Tell the patients how they use us as guinea pigs or experimental monkeys!"[40] Further experiments are carried out on prisoners and people who are homeless, many "who came from the county hospital and jail, both men and women," and "didn't know exactly what kind of treatment they were receiving."[41] As his own health improves, Contreras indeed sees something predatory happening to those around him, and he becomes more attuned to the radical critique emerging from those politically marginalized in the hospital and beyond.

If memory in *The Captain* operates as I suggest—that is, as a narrative device—the novel also shows how cultural texts in the twenty-first century can restage official histories as contested, as always already negotiating refusal and resistance as counterhegemonic responses. This refusal is perhaps most evident in the character Sandro Díez, an incarcerated patient at Olive View who seeks to disrupt the fantasy of the sanatorium as a benevolent institution. Rather, Díez sees a carceral operation with economic and political agendas. A former Pacific Pipe Clay and Cement Company employee with "a reputation of being a subversive, political or social troublemaker," he insists to Contreras that he be allowed to narrate his own position as an exploited, racialized radical laborer, and to be represented as such in the *Point*.[42] Díez is admitted to Olive View after the company doctor claims he has been infected with tuberculosis. He tells Contreras that he rejected the diagnosis and, after momentarily resisting Díez's version of what happened with the doctors, finally agrees to write an account of Díez's arrest and incarceration for the *Point*. In it, he recounts the arrest and detainment of his family, who are also labeled as contagious TB carriers, explaining that the real motivation behind their arrest had to do with Díez's subversive politics as a union organizer. The Pacific Pipe Clay and Cement Company's exploitative and abusive working conditions drive Díez to unsuccessfully seek help from the other workers and their union: "They listened to me but were too afraid for their jobs to act. It took something ugly to make them finally respond."[43] He initiates a protest after seeing another beating, a sexual assault, and other commonplace acts of violence. His actions, Díez insists, prompt the company to use quarantine laws as a tool to incarcerate, but what astonishes him most is the fact that such violence is sanctioned and unexceptional. Public displays of violence at the clay yard are represented as ongoing, mundane spectacles—the foreman smashing "his fist into the woman's face," yet Díez recognizes that it would take "something ugly to make them finally respond." The connection between the hospital and the prison is made explicit in this scene, and Díez claims that, for him, "the sanatorium is jail. I'm not being treated here. I'm being punished! I'm a political prisoner because I suffer from a political disease!"[44]

Díez's fictionalized narrative is likely based on an actual event. In an interview recorded in 1996, Morales refers to a conversation he had about someone's family incarceration at a hospital: "A man came to me about [my earlier novels]. He mentioned . . . how sometimes in the 1950s Chicanos were disappearing, and I asked, 'What do you mean disappearing? Were they being deported?' and he said, 'No, no, no. They took my dad and my brothers and me away, and they said that we had tuberculosis. They took us here, to the county hospital in Orange County, and they held us for about a year. But we were never sick.'" Morales pressed the man for details, and he continued: "'They thought we were some kind of political radicals and that we were organizing certain unions and doing this and that. So that was a way of taking us out of circulation.'"[45] As a cultural text, *The Captain* documents an archival experience through the memories of those who were "gathered for experimental surgery," who "signed waivers without even knowing how to read," and, perhaps most difficult to navigate, those whose stories were nowhere to be found in the archive or official records.

What does a meditation on memory such as this tell us about what is missing and what is absent? Here, in that tension between fiction and history, is where we might locate an important engagement with the historical framing of medical technologies. These fictional characters recognize this distinction between official history and a more collective memory as a narrative tug that frames their story as one with political stakes and historical importance. The everyday lives of the people in the sanatorium, as Contreras in his later years comes to understand, ought to be documented: "Almost fifty years later [after Olive View] I would read the fascinating and little-known history of this beautiful place in a thesis my great-nephew . . . wrote while he was a medical student at the University of California, Los Angeles. In Olive View's history, Gregory deciphered the sanatorium's mystical, romantic, and frightful dimensions and how they intersected with its staff's, doctors', and patients' lives. . . . Gregory considered my life, like Olive View's history, important and valuable enough to be recorded and saved in his study."[46] If "knowing the history of these buildings sheds a completely different perspective on what having tuberculosis was and meant," what medicine represents on a cultural front and as a politics of representation is the critical capacity not only to examine "how medicine became abusive" but also to interrogate the narratives of medical progress and the possessiveness of knowledge, how it is always already racialized and gendered, and what is at stake in remembering what is easily forgotten.[47]

Futures of Medical Violence

On November 24, 2010, Barack Obama asked the Presidential Commission for the Study of Bioethical Issues to review regulations for domestic and international standards on experimental scientific and medical research involving protections for human subjects. The request followed a chance discovery in John C. Cutler's papers at the University of Pittsburgh after a historian stumbled on records of covert scientific experiments.[1] Conducted under the supervision of the United States Public Health Service (USPHS), the papers documented the deliberate transmission of syphilis to people in prisons and hospitals in Guatemala City from 1946 to 1948. For over two years, scientists carried out deadly and dangerous trials on imprisoned men, soldiers, sex workers, and children in an orphanage, finding wards of the state and human subjects they deemed to be usable for the production of knowledge and for the progress of medicine. To better understand the transmission of syphilis and gonorrhea, the doctors exposed over 1,300 people, most of whom were under various forms of captivity and coercion, to these contagious diseases. They were infected through old and new procedures, sometimes by the more traditional modes of directly rubbing mixtures into the skin (similar to those methods practice by Edward Arning in the 1880s) and into open sores and around the genital areas and by coerced and forced semisurgical operations, in some cases on children. Other methods involved hiring sex workers to have sex with imprisoned men and to conscript soldiers in military barracks. Less than half of the people who were exposed received treatments after contracting a disease, with the untreated used as a control to measure against others who did receive treatment. Many suffered the physical pain of the experiments and the pain caused by the development of syphilis in the body. Many people, including descendants of the medical subjects, died prematurely as a result.

This story echoes another. The well-rehearsed and still-contested story of Tuskegee is one site of continuous questioning.[2] Susan Reverby, an established historian of the Tuskegee syphilis experiments, suggests that many issues complicate the telling of what happened there but in particular that popular notions of how infectious disease is spread in scientific experiments tend to be enmeshed in complex sets of truths, fictions, and fantasies. Narrating contested histories constitutes not only informing publics about what occurred and to whom but also conveying the minutiae of science under scrutiny—in particular, its practices and procedures. That part is particularly difficult because it requires explaining how "doctors could not just inject the spirochetal bacteria that cause syphilis easily from the blood of one person to another."[3] Centuries of such supposed experimental research demonstrates another set of explanatory challenges, as well as the opportunities presented by trying to recreate various diseases in uninfected, otherwise healthy bodies. This, says the refrain of scientific authority, is the hard work of experts, not for laypeople to challenge, question, or doubt. Indeed, beyond syphilis, other contagious diseases such as gonorrhea, tuberculosis, and Hansen's disease provided scientists and doctors lifelong careers based on the problem of locating infectious disease and identifying the causes of transmission, the potential for inoculation, and the promise of cures. Anyone looking to understand the story of Tuskegee, and other kinds of medical violence such as those discussed in this book, is confronted with the immense time commitment of learning the science of medicine, grasping the implemented practices of public health, and navigating how multiple communities, institutions, and the people within them have the narrative power to define what happens in order to achieve the kind of supposed progress that truly benefits the public. And if this was meant to be a covert project, the truer way to understand it is that it was a public and open secret—in Harriet Washington's phrasing, hidden in plain view.[4]

When Cutler's forgotten archives resurfaced, the United States government seemed to embrace the moment of righting an obvious wrong. Secretary of State Hillary Clinton and Secretary of the Department of Health and Human Services (HHS) Kathleen Sebelius released a public statement that apologized to the people and government of Guatemala and, in English and Spanish, denounced the experiments as illegitimate, anomalous, and reprehensible behavior carried out "under the guise of public health."[5] The complete statement reads:

The sexually transmitted disease inoculation study conducted from 1946–1948 in Guatemala was clearly unethical. Although these events occurred more than 64 years ago, we are outraged that such reprehensible research could have occurred under the guise of public health. We deeply regret that it happened, and we apologize to all the individuals who were affected by such abhorrent research practices. The conduct exhibited during the study does not represent the values of the United States, or our commitment to human dignity and great respect for the people of Guatemala. The study is a sad reminder that adequate human subject safeguards did not exist a half-century ago.

Today, the regulations that govern U.S.-funded human medical research prohibit these kinds of appalling violations. The United States is unwavering in our commitment to ensure that all human medical studies conducted today meet exacting U.S. and international legal and ethical standards. In the spirit of this commitment to ethical research, we are launching a thorough investigation into the specifics of this case from 1946. In addition, through the Presidential Commission for the Study of Bioethical Issues, we are also convening a body of international experts to review and report on the most effective methods to ensure that all human medical research conducted around the globe today meets rigorous ethical standards.

The people of Guatemala are our close friends and neighbors in the Americas. Our countries partner together on a range of issues, and our people are bound together by shared values, commerce, and by the many Guatemalan Americans who enrich our country. As we move forward to better understand this appalling event, we reaffirm the importance of our relationship with Guatemala, and our respect for the Guatemalan people, as well as our commitment to the highest standards of ethics in medical research.[6]

What, exactly, are the terms of this public and official apology? Although the study occurred over sixty years before—within the temporality of the statement, an eternity—the progress of medical science in that current moment could not imagine such events. It was both "reprehensible" and a mockery of actual research, not legitimate work but the epitome of bad science. And yet it happened, with deep regret, under the supervision of the Public Health Service. As a problem to manage in the political present, the official apology raises the level of accountability and signals to people across the globe that such conduct, unequivocally, "does not represent the values of the United States." Instead it demonstrates the "sad reminder" that the past was either unconcerned with the protection of human medical subjects or unenlightened about the value and necessity of protecting human life— especially the most vulnerable to exploitation, violation, and harm or premature death. Rather than rationalize the research and distance from blame—the tendency of the following Trump administration—the Obama administration walked a careful line that conveyed an ethical approach to a state-sanctioned act of predatory medicine and public health. What developed around the discovery of the cache of medical records appeared to be an awareness of the high stakes of how the experiment should be remembered. It also sought an avenue of moral capability and credibility that not only relied on political narrative but looked to the analysis and evaluation of medical researchers and historians, bioethicists and human rights experts, legalists, and others— those who ultimately constituted the Presidential Commission for the Study of Bioethical Issues. The charge of the president called to service a group of experts to tell the public how serious this discovery was and how seriously the administration took it.

President Obama quickly initiated conversations with Guatemalan President Álvaro Colom on October 1, 2010, during which he issued a personal apology for these U.S.-led medical experiments. The news media covered President Obama's expressions of "deep regret" for the unethical research and his "unwavering commitment" to ensure that such human medical studies would not occur in the present. Current transnational medical research sanctioned by the United States would more than ever prioritize the protection of its human subjects over its institutions and value the dignity of people involved over its officials and its reputation.[7] In concert with the president's personal apology, Clinton and Sebelius issued an official apology to the people and government of Guatemala, acknowledging that the United States organized and funded the medical experiments.[8] They described the experiments as "clearly unethical" but then quickly focused the discussion on maintaining international trade and labor relations with Guatemala. Naming the people of Guatemala as "our close friends and neighbors in the Americas," the statement concludes by noting that the two countries' history of collaboration is tethered by "shared values, commerce, and by the many Guatemalan Americans who enrich our country." When faced with how to narrate the humanitarian visions of medical work and values, represented in this context by the USPHS, the question of how to deliver this history reveals major contradictions that are not able to be worked out within the logics of liberal humanitarianism. That is, the apology, as a statement, must distance itself from the very actions it sanctions, as Secretaries Clinton and Sebelius insist that the "conduct exhibited during the study does not represent the values of the United States."

While sifting through John C. Cutler's Tuskegee Study of Untreated Syphilis papers at the University of Pittsburgh, Reverby accidentally stumbled on a cache of records that documented covert syphilis experiments in Guatemala City.[9] The project was funded and conducted by U.S. Public Health Service doctors from 1946 to 1948. As a high-ranking U.S. Public Health Service medical officer, Cutler's human-based research took him to Guatemala, India, and Haiti. He supervised experiments on incarcerated people at Terre Haute and Sing Sing prisons and joined the Tuskegee syphilis experiments in the 1960s.[10] After serving as assistant surgeon general in 1958, Cutler was offered a professorship at the University of Pittsburgh. After a lifetime of impunity carrying out acts that would be criminalized in most other circumstances, the highly respected scientist ended his academic career as dean of the Graduate School of Public Health in the 1990s.

Cutler was in no way an anomaly or rogue scientist in medicine. Rather, he was representative of how mainstream scientific discourse has been conducted for years—generally behind closed doors and with the authority and resources of the state, universities, hospitals, and laboratories.[11] Documents in Cutler's archives reveal caches of letters, notes, reports, photographs, and official correspondences between doctors in Guatemala and the United States showing that what was occurring was understood as acceptable and legitimate science. Very little in them suggests that such experimentation was anomalous. What is clear, however, is that scientists and the United States Public Health Service worked to keep the covert trials and research from the general public. The great lengths state-supported efforts took to normalize submission and coercion are widely documented during the time. The United States funded covert operations in the 1940s intended to destabilize the Guatemalan government, creating the conditions for the closed-door operations understood as U.S. intervention and opening up other kinds of possibilities for science.[12] In the words of Cutler, speaking as the lead scientist of the Guatemala syphilis study: "It was deemed advisable, from the point of view of public and personnel relations, to work so that as few people as possible know the experimental procedure."[13]

Indeed, G. Robert Coatney—a renowned USPHS malaria expert who, in the decades following, would be widely praised for his groundbreaking work in tropical medicine—wrote to Cutler about the experiments, noting his casual conversations with leading doctors about their frustrations with stifled attempts to conduct such experimental work in the United States. Coatney mentions in a letter to Cutler that one of the doctors was acting U.S. Surgeon General Thomas Parran, about whom Coatney notes: "As you well know, [Parran] is very much interested in the project and a merry twinkle came into his eye when he said, 'You know, we couldn't do such an experiment in this country.'"[14] Cutler was advised by his supervisors in the United States to forgo consent discussions with Indigenous Mayan prisoners because they were "only confused by explanations and knowing what is happening." While U.S. and Guatemalan authorities worked together to create these conditions and to inoculate prisoner-patients, asylum patients, and children in orphanages, most were not informed of the nature of the experiments and never gave consent to do so. Guatemalan doctors and government officials made possible the site of experimentation, and as several exchanges occurred to facilitate it, the praise and encouragement of figures like Cutler came from all directions. In a letter from Dr. Roberto Robles Chinchille to the "Distinguished Dr. Cutler," the director of medical services at the Penitenciaría Central de Guatemala spoke on behalf of the incarcerated subjects to express an unconditional gratitude: "It is a privilege for us, to manifest you, by means of this lines, [*sic*] our everlasting gratitude which will remain for ever in our hearts, because of your noble and gentlemanly way with which you have alleviated the suffering of the guards, and prisoners of this penitentiary."[15] The letter was cited in Cutler's 1955 report on the experiments.

Reverby published the discovery of the archive in a journal in January of 2010, but only after she urged a former director of the Centers for Disease Control (CDC) to pressure the agency to investigate did they begin to respond. When the statement hit the public and the press covered the story, outrage on both political and medical fronts took the spotlight. In the *New York Times,* Dr. Mark Siegler, director of the MacLean Center for Clinical Medical Ethics at the University of Chicago's medical school, is quoted as saying: "It's ironic—no, it's worse than that, it's appalling—that, at the same time as the United States was prosecuting Nazi doctors for crimes against humanity, the U.S. government was supporting research that placed human subjects at enormous risk."[16] Bioethicists asked repeatedly how this could happen, raising questions about reparations to survivors and descendants, what the United States owes the Guatemalan government (even as the Guatemalan government facilitated those experiments), and who might be accountable for these "abhorrent research practices." For a moment, this historical event represented what one medical expert dubbed "a dark chapter in the history of medicine."[17]

While experts, policy makers, and media outlets, among others, were astonished by the uncovering of these documents because they appeared new, unthinkable, and anomalous, this "dark chapter" of medical history is deliberately and deeply embedded into the infrastructure and formation of Western medicine. As *Archiving Medical Violence* has attempted to show, human experimentation on and medical mistreatment of racialized, disenfranchised people in prisons, hospital wards, sanatoriums, orphanages, the military, colonies, sex work, and beyond has been the fuel of medical progress. As scientist Edward Arning repeatedly suggested (discussed in chapter 1), these are the conditions of possibility, the raw materials, of medical knowledge, done to serve a greater good. The story of criminalized Indigenous people and people of color in the medical archive has long been a guiding narrative of scientific advancement, even if unacknowledged in official discourse. While situated as something like rogue science, the narration of these medical records in the media pulls from other chapters of medicine to make sense of it, such as the medical experiments of Nazi scientists, the Tuskegee syphilis experiments, and others, because they not only resonate with experimentation in Guatemala but are directly connected to it. The so-called research was a continuous body of work that produced many narratives that traveled across multiple terrains through public and private forms of print culture to contain contagious diseases.

One of the terms of the Obama administration's apology, then, is the ongoing effort to provincialize the medicalized past. That statement outlines several questions at the heart of this book, which takes as its focal point the problem of medical violence as subsumed by the narratives of medical progress, humanitarianism, and benevolence. Those experiments were carried out by world-renowned and highly respected scientists and government agents, yet the tone of the 2010 statement seems to leave little room for misinterpretation about the ethical and moral concerns of the project designed to expand knowledge for the public good. In a letter by President Obama to the chair of the Presidential Commission for the Study of Bioethical Issues, the request to review the policies for "human subject protections" takes center stage. The end of the letter offers commentary on the present state of human subject research, why and how the investigation should proceed, and future implications. President Obama's statement reads:

> While I believe the research community has made tremendous progress in the area of human subject protection, what took place in Guatemala is a *sobering reminder of past abuses.* It is especially important for the Commission to use its vast expertise spanning the fields of science, policy, ethics, and religious values to carry out this mission. We owe it to the people of Guatemala *and future generations of volunteers who participate in medical research.*[18]

In one reading, the faith that U.S. researchers working within and beyond U.S. borders have "made tremendous progress" in the realm of human subject protections remains stable and unshaken. The narrative of progress underlying the statement requires such faith in the state project focused not only on notions of a national public good but also on global ethics. Even as the discovery makes visible a kind of subterranean logic of medical knowledge production—one that operates through a racial hierarchy of white supremacy, racial capitalism, and settler colonialism—the voice of the nation doubles down on the investments of scientific benevolence. Read closely, Obama's statement tempers that unwavering confidence with other gestures, which offer a condition of possibility for such progress narratives to hold into the future. That medical experimentation in Guatemala represents a "sobering reminder of past abuses" is an important reproduction of how the nation actively holds violence in a static past. It is in memory, as a reminder, that the formation of violence can be articulated. It is a guide for modifying the present as opposed to the context for the present, what the United States owes to not only "the people of Guatemala" but also to "the future generations of volunteers who participate in medical research." The imperative to maintain a medical future of the state, grounded in moral claims that require a language of social debt and humanitarianism, is imagined as a figure of, at once, the violated (in this specific instance, the Guatemalan subjects and family survivors) and the violator (state-managed scientific research). When these archives surfaced in 2010, U.S. representatives and human rights advocates quickly condemned the acts these documents record; yet situating those archives complicates a narration of history. Survivors and family members attempted to hold the United States accountable through the court system, but the U.S. District Courts ruled in 2013 that the United States was protected from lawsuits under two separate immunity laws: the Federal Tort Claims Act and the International Organizations Immunities Act.[19] In 2015, lawsuits representing victims, family members, and others against Johns Hopkins were again rejected. In a statement to the Johns Hopkins University community, along with a media statement with similar sentiment, Ronald J. Daniels (president of John Hopkins University), Paul B. Rothman (dean of the medical faculty and CEO of Johns Hopkins Medicine), and Michael J. Klag (dean of Johns Hopkins Bloomberg School of Public Health) declared: "This was not a Johns Hopkins study. Johns Hopkins did not initiate, pay for, direct or conduct the study in Guatemala. Participation in the review of government research was then and is today separate from being a Johns Hopkins employee, and no nonprofit university or hospital has ever been held liable for a study conducted by the U.S. government."[20] Only recently have those suits been reinstated, although not without serious counterefforts by those in the medical establishment. Even as that conversation shifted with a civil lawsuit in 2017 under the Alien Tort Statute, the courts would find that Johns Hopkins University could be held responsible as a private, rather than a government, entity.

I want to highlight how this rhetorical move conjures the past and the future as the specter of medical violence. Like the story of violence writ large, Obama's statement signals the fugitive subject that constitutes an unruly state archive and yet-to-be-determined generations of willing bodies for medical progress. The discovery of this study adds to a long list of U.S.-sanctioned research conducted in the name of progress, several of which I analyze in the previous chapters, but what does the management of medical violence reveal about the racial state, the conditions of impossibility of consent, and those alternate medical futures seeking to reimagine the terms of justice? How are the terms of ethics worked out under a medical imperative that, at once, protects one supposed public while killing another—in which the publics cut across contested narrative spaces of race, gender, sexuality, coloniality, ability, locality, and body politics? Under what conditions does medical violence navigate its own institutional presence in, for instance, hospitals, prisons, quarantine settlements, plantations, occupied lands, borderlands, and migrant labor camps, but also in and through national and international law and policy designed to govern those spaces, institutions, and discourses? And what does this mean as a project of history, memory, and culture? Put another way, what are the terms of the past under medical violence? *Archiving Medical Violence* presses on medical narratives existing in tension with those of the state to assert that the reexamination of the institutions and archives of public health and public security—particularly their multiple registers—points to how narratives of medicine work to mediate state imperatives. In their most effective manifestation, such archives subsume violence into narratives of modern reason, progress, and law. Definitions of state-sanctioned violence are "either lawmaking or law preserving," while violence perceived outside these parameters "forfeits all validity."[21] It is therefore understood in such articulations as antagonistic or as criminal to the state. And yet in a medical imagination, violence clearly inhabits other locations, as one influential scientist casually observes when asked about the state's relationship to medical experimentation: "Well, . . . it's against the law to do many things, but the law winks when a reputable man wants to do a scientific experiment."[22]

How do such sites continue to unsettle narratives that forget in the name of national imperatives? How do they produce those national narratives as ahistorical by subsuming their own violent pasts? What I examine in this study, then, are the conditions for the law's "wink"—the state management of medical violence as a continuum, overwhelmingly made up of devalued subjects who are revalued under necropolitical imperatives to protect some by sanctioning death for others. Memory and forgetting work to produce and firm up national meaning as much as they provide the possibility for shifting and reshaping it. In this context, looking to cultural memory might prompt questioning "why and how we remember—for what purpose, for whom, and from which position we remember—even when discussing sites of memory, where to many the significance of remembering seems obvious."[23]

NOTES

Preface and Acknowledgments

1. Saidiya Hartman, "The Death Toll," in *The Quarantine Files: Thinkers in Self-Isolation,* ed. Brad Evans (Los Angeles: Los Angeles Review of Books, 2020), https://lareviewofbooks.org/article/quarantine-files-thinkers-self-isolation/.

2. Megan L. Ranney, Valerie Griffeth, and Ashish K. Jha, "Critical Supply Shortages: The Need for Ventilators and Personal Protective Equipment during the Covid-19 Pandemic," *New England Journal of Medicine* 382, no. 18 (2020): e41, https://doi.org/10.1056/NEJMp2006141.

3. "WHO Coronavirus (COVID-19) Dashboard," World Health Organization, accessed January 13, 2023, https://covid19.who.int/?mapFilter=deaths.

Introduction

1. *UnSeen: Our Past in a New Light, Ken Gonzales-Day and Titus Kaphar,* Smithsonian National Portrait Gallery, May 31, 2018–January 6, 2019, https://npg.si.edu/about-us/press-release/national-portrait-gallery-presents-"unseen-our-past-new-light-ken-gonzales.

2. I draw on works by Lisa Lowe, Roderick Ferguson, Saidiya Hartman, Sylvia Wynter, Jodi Melamed, and others to point to how archives, and narratives underpinning them, make possible the enactment and elision of multiple forms of violence.

3. Macarena Gómez-Barris notes that, in national projects taking up their own histories of colonialism and state violence, culture has been "a key arena of the selective management of colonial history toward producing a stable national culture in unstable times." Macarena Gómez-Barris, *Where Memory Dwells: Culture and State Violence in Chile* (Berkeley: University of California Press, 2009), 1.

4. For recent analyses of Trump-era social movements, see Naomi Paik, *Borders, Walls, Raids, Sanctuary: Understanding U.S. Immigration for the Twenty-First Century* (Berkeley: University of California Press, 2020); Julie Sze, *Environmental Justice in a Moment of Danger* (Berkeley: University of California Press, 2020).

5. Eve Tuck and K. Wayne Yang, "Introduction: Born Under the Rising Sign

of Social Justice," in *Toward What Justice? Describing Diverse Dreams of Justice in Education,* ed. Eve Tuck and K. Wayne Yang, 1–17 (New York: Routledge, 2018).

6. Ken Gonzales-Day, "Installation View of *Unseen: Our Past in a New Light,* at the NPG, Smithsonian," https://kengonzalesday.com/projects/profiled-series/. Tyler Green, Ken Gonzales-Day, and Rachel Conrad, "No. 498: Ken Gonzales-Day, Tony Conrad," May 20, 2021, in *Modern Art Notes Podcast,* produced by Tyler Green, podcast, MP3 audio, 1:13:59, https://manpodcast.com/portfolio/no-498-ken-gonzales-day-tony-conrad/.

7. In *Lynching in the West,* Gonzales-Day also notes that taking stock of what digitization of archives opens has the potential to change the way information can be organized in the future. He further considers "the impact of the institutional, regional, and subject archives and their reliance upon the copy print in shaping historical awareness—and this issue is of increasing interest as an expanding number of institutions begin to digitize their material holdings. In practice, the backs of photographic images are almost never reproduced as either copy prints or digital files, a logistical reality that in the case of lynching photographs can also lead to the loss of information, such as a handwritten note across the back. Digital libraries and archives are some of the fastest growing resources in the nation, and questions of metadata coding provide an amazing opportunity to rethink the very categories, or values, traditionally assigned to a given media, digital technology can also provide new levels of access and potentially draw attention to new properties of the source object." Ken Gonzales-Day, *Lynching in the West, 1850–1935* (Durham, N.C.: Duke University Press, 2006), 202.

8. Saidiya Hartman, *Scenes of Subjection: Terror, Slavery, and Self-Making in Nineteenth-Century America* (New York: Oxford University Press, 1997); Judith Butler, *Precarious Life: The Powers of Mourning and Violence* (London: Verso, 2006).

9. Iyko Day highlights the importance of the landscape as a framing device, noting that as life-size representations hanging in museums, Gonzales-Day's *Erased Lynching* series ultimately inserts viewers into the scene, "implicating us as consumers of the spectacle of racial violence and participants in their circulation." My reading diverges in that the emphasis is less about interacting with or becoming part of the mob ("implicating us as consumers of the spectacle") than it is about flipping the "wonder gaze" of the mob onto itself. In other words, the very removal of the body highlights the lynch mob as the (always already) spectacle. Iyko Day, *Alien Capital: Asian Racialization and the Logic of Settler Colonial Capitalism* (Durham, N.C.: Duke University Press, 2016), 75.

10. Nicole M. Guidotti-Hernández, *Unspeakable Violence: Remapping U.S. and Mexican National Imaginaries* (Durham, N.C.: Duke University Press, 2011), 5. Guidotti-Hernández elaborates on the representational politics of historizing racial violence: "The story I tell is not a happy one, yet there is a graciousness to the intervention I'm trying to make. I take up my case studies because

they have been or easily could be part of a resistance narrative, the very thing I cautiously try not to reproduce. Hence, I make three basic arguments that unseat and question resistance narratives: first, there is a disjuncture between the celebratory narratives of mestizaje (social, racial, and cultural hybridity as a form of the Spanish colonial collision with Indians in the Americas) and hybridity that compose Mexican, Chicana/o, and other nationalisms and the literally unspeakable violence that characterized the borderlands in the nineteenth century and the early twentieth. Second, violence is and was the one factor that determined how racial positioning, gender, and class alliances played themselves out in contests over citizenship and resources. Third, the formalistic reporting of these events follows a similar pattern of using repetition as a way of denying violence as a foundation of national history, making these events unspeakable" (4).

11. Guidotti-Hernández, *Unspeakable Violence,* 5. See also Hartman, *Scenes of Subjection;* Gonzales-Day, *Lynching in the West;* Koritha Mitchell, *Living with Lynching: African American Lynching Plays, Performance, and Citizenship, 1890–1930* (Champaign: University of Illinois Press, 2011); Fred Moten, *In the Break: The Aesthetics of the Black Radical Tradition* (Minneapolis: University of Minnesota Press, 2003).

12. Guidotti-Hernández, *Unspeakable Violence,* 8–9.

13. Mitchell, *Living with Lynching,* 1–3. "In these photographs, a crowd typically surrounds the 'criminal' it has subdued, and the corpse is often still hanging from a tree, telephone pole, or bridge. Yet during the same decades in which these pictures were originally created and distributed, African Americans wrote plays about mob violence that tell stories strikingly different from those suggested by lynching photography." Mitchell continues: "When real-life lynchings became theatrical, whites literally used *pieces* of black bodies as props to perform their *master* status. In other words, African Americans viewed lynching as a theater of mastery in which whites seeking (not assuming) racial supremacy used the black body as muse, antagonist, and stage prop. The vengeance with which some whites performed their supposedly superior status is quite revealing. As cultural theorists have long contended, hegemony is never complete; it must continually reassert itself. Thus, if white supremacists denied black humanity, black familial ties, and achievement, African Americans must have been convincingly establishing it" (3).

14. See Titus Kaphar, *Behind the Myth of Benevolence,* 2014 (oil on canvas, 59 × 34 × 7 inches), https://www.kapharstudio.com/behind-the-myth-of-benevolence/.

15. See Toni Morrison, *Playing in the Dark: Whiteness and the Literary Imagination* (Cambridge, Mass.: Harvard University Press, 1992); Robert Warrior, "'The Finest Men We Have Ever Seen': Reading Jefferson's Osage Encounters through *Orientalism,*" *ARIEL: A Review of International English Literature* 51, no. 1 (January 2020): 57–80.

16. See Marita Sturken, *Tangled Memories: The Vietnam War, the AIDS*

Epidemic, and the Politics of Remembering (Berkeley: University of California Press, 1997); Lisa Yoneyama, *Hiroshima Traces: Time, Space, and the Dialectics of Memory* (Berkeley: University of California Press, 1999). For a compelling reading of national memory and white supremacist violence as a rupture in the present, framed by recent movements at Standing Rock and at Charlottesville, see Warrior, "'The Finest Men We Have Ever Seen.'"

17. Nicholas Mirzoeff, *The Right to Look: A Counterhistory of Visuality* (Durham, N.C.: Duke University Press, 2011).

18. Chandan Reddy, *Freedom with Violence: Race, Sexuality, and the US State* (Durham, N.C.: Duke University Press, 2011); Jodi Melamed, *Represent and Destroy: Racializing Violence in the New Racial Capitalism* (Minneapolis: University of Minnesota Press, 2003).

19. Sylvia Wynter, "Unsettling the Coloniality of Being/Power/Truth/Freedom: Towards the Human, After Man, Its Overrepresentation—An Argument," *CR: The New Centennial Review* 3, no. 3 (Fall 2003): 257–337; Denise Ferreira da Silva, "Before *Man*: Sylvia Wynter's Rewriting of the Modern Episteme," in *Sylvia Wynter: On Being Human as Praxis*, ed. Katherine McKittrick, 90–105 (Durham, N.C.: Duke University Press, 2015); Walter D. Mignolo, "Sylvia Wynter: What Does It Mean to Be Human?," in *Sylvia Wynter: On Being Human as Praxis*, ed. Katherine McKittrick, 106–23 (Durham, N.C.: Duke University Press, 2015).

20. Melamed, *Represent and Destroy*, 2.

21. Lisa Lowe provides an important definitional frame for my interrogations of culture: "Culture is the medium of the *present*—the imagined equivalences and identifications through which the individual invents lived relationship with the national collective—but it is simultaneously the site that mediates the *past*, through which history is grasped as difference, as fragments, shocks, and flashes of disjunction. It is through culture that the subject becomes, acts, and speaks itself as 'American.' It is likewise in culture that individuals and collectivities struggle and remember and, in that difficult remembering, imagine and practice both subject and community differently." Lisa Lowe, *Immigrant Acts: On Asian American Cultural Politics* (Durham, N.C.: Duke University Press, 1996), 2. Melamed highlights literary studies as one of the foremost cultural technologies for "producing, transmitting, and implanting official antiracist knowledges." Melamed, *Represent and Destroy*, 15. In this role, literary studies has come to play a uniquely powerful part in producing commonsense notions about race in the United States after World War II, for better or worse. It is important to stress that literary texts themselves are not at issue here, rather literary studies as materially produced discourses.

22. Over two decades of contributions to medical cultural studies, history, and science and technology studies have engaged significant conversations anchored in questions of race, sexuality, colonialism, white supremacy, citizenship, and representation. Significant to this study: Dorothy Roberts, *Killing the Black Body: Race, Reproduction, and the Meaning of Liberty* (New York: Ran-

dom House, 2008); Nayan Shah, *Contagious Divides: Epidemics and Race in San Francisco's Chinatown* (Berkeley: University of California Press, 2001); Warwick Anderson, *Colonial Pathologies: American Tropical Medicine, Race, and Hygiene in the Philippines* (Durham, N.C.: Duke University Press, 2006); Natalia Molina, *Fit to Be Citizens? Public Health and Race in Los Angeles, 1879–1939* (Berkeley: University of California Press, 2006); Priscilla Wald, *Contagious: Cultures, Carriers, and the Outbreak Narrative* (Durham, N.C.: Duke University Press, 2008); Harriet A. Washington, *Medical Apartheid: The Dark History of Medical Experimentation on Black Americans from Colonial Times to the Present* (New York: Random House, 2008); Ruha Benjamin, *People's Science: Bodies and Rights on the Stem Cell Frontier* (Berkeley: University of California Press, 2006); Kerri Inglis, *Maʻi Lepera: Disease and Displacement in Nineteenth-Century Hawaiʻi* (Honolulu: University of Hawaiʻi Press, 2013); Kim TallBear, *Native American DNA*; Alexandra Minna Stern, *Eugenic Nation: Faults and Frontiers of Better Breeding in Modern America* (Berkeley: University of California Press, 2015); Neel Ahuja, *Bioinsecurities: Disease Interventions, Empire, and the Government of Species* (Durham, N.C.: Duke University Press, 2016); Ruha Benjamin, ed., *Captivating Technology: Race, Carceral Technoscience, and Liberatory Imagination in Everyday Life* (Durham, N.C.: Duke University Press, 2019).

23. Michelle Moran, *Colonizing Leprosy: Imperialism and the Politics of Public Health in the United States* (Chapel Hill: University of North Carolina Press, 2012).

24. Stern, *Eugenic Nation*; Alexandra Minna Stern, "Buildings, Boundaries, and Blood: Medicalization and Nation-Building on the U.S.–Mexico Border, 1910–1930," *Hispanic American Historical Review* 79, no. 1 (1999): 41–81; Kelly Lytle Hernández, *Migra! A History of the U.S. Border Patrol* (Berkeley: University of California Press, 2010).

25. Avery Gordon, *Ghostly Matters: Haunting and the Sociological Imagination* (Minneapolis: University of Minnesota Press, 2008); Avery Gordon, *The Hawthorn Archive: Letters from the Utopian Margins* (New York: Fordham University Press, 2017); Saidiya Hartman, *Wayward Lives, Beautiful Experiments: Intimate Histories of Riotous Black Girls, Troublesome Women, and Queer Radicals* (New York: Norton, 2019); Jodi Kim, *Ends of Empire: Asian American Critique and the Cold War* (Minneapolis: University of Minnesota Press, 2010); Lisa Lowe, *The Intimacies of Four Continents* (Durham, N.C.: Duke University Press, 2015); Tiya Miles, *Ties That Bind: The Story of an Afro-Cherokee Family in Slavery and Freedom*, 2nd ed. (Berkeley: University of California Press, 2015); Ann Laura Stoler, *Haunted by Empire: Geographies of Intimacy in North American History* (Durham, N.C.: Duke University Press, 2006).

26. Lowe argues for understanding "archives of liberalism" as a model for analyzing economies of "affirmation and forgetting" that structures and formalizes in official archives of "liberalism, and liberal ways of understanding." The notion of freedom for "man," as defined by European and North American

philosophical frameworks, at the same time relegates others to "geographical and temporal spaces that are constituted as backward, uncivilized, and unfree." The model is particularly useful for reading narratives of freedom made possible by forgetting, denying, or erasing colonial slavery, Indigenous dispossession, and displaced peoples across continents. It problematizes the notion that social inequality is resolvable through rights discourse defined by groups categorized as fully "human," while at the same time locating other subjects, practices, and geographies "at a distance from 'the human.'" Lowe, *Intimacies of Four Continents*, 3–4.

27. Lowe, *Immigrant Acts*, 2.

28. Lisa Lowe and David Lloyd, *The Politics of Culture in the Shadow of Capital* (Durham, N.C.: Duke University Press, 2006), 1.

29. On sanctioned violence, see Giorgio Agamben, *Homo Sacer: Sovereign Power and Bare Life*, trans. Daniel Heller-Roazen (Stanford, Calif.: Stanford University Press, 1998), 156.

30. Kalindi Vora, *Life Support: Biocapital and the New History of Outsourced Labor* (Minneapolis: University of Minnesota Press, 2015), 20.

31. Vora, *Life Support*, 3.

32. For discussions about the politics of museums and state archives, see Sandy Grande, Natalie Avalos, Jason Mancini, Christopher Newell, and endawnis Spears, "Red Praxis: Lessons from Mashantucket to Standing Rock," in *Standing with Standing Rock: Voices from the #NODAPL Movement*, eds. Nick Estes and Jaskiran Dhillon (Minneapolis: University of Minnesota, 2019); Sandy Grande, *Red Pedagogy: Native American Social and Political Thought* (Lanham, Md.: Rowman and Littlefield, 2015); Lisa Lowe, "History Hesitant," *Social Text* (125) 33, no. 4 (December 2015): 85–107.

33. Tuck and Yang, "Introduction."

34. I am paraphrasing Roderick Ferguson's formulation, which theorizes queer of color analysis as critique that "presumes that liberal ideology occludes the intersecting saliency of race, gender, sexuality, and class in forming social practices. Approaching ideologies of transparency as formations that have worked to conceal those intersections means that queer of color analysis has to debunk the idea that race, class, gender, and sexuality are discrete formations, apparently insulated from one another. As queer of color critique challenges ideologies of discreteness, it attempts to disturb the idea that racial and national formations are obviously disconnected." Roderick Ferguson, *Aberrations in Black: Toward a Queer of Color Critique* (Minneapolis: University of Minnesota Press, 2004), 4.

35. Originally commissioned by HBO and Oprah Winfrey as part of the marketing and promotion of the 2017 feature film about Lacks, the portrait depicts a woman both life-size and larger-than-life. This story was reintroduced to mainstream imaginaries by Rebecca Skloot's 2010 best-selling book, before being elevated as a feature film through HBO. At the start of the twenty-first

century, Lacks's story produced new life that resonated as an unexplained crisis of medicine, even as that crisis had been present for centuries and was felt across the public and intimate spheres of race, gender, sexuality, and personhood. See Harriett Washington's seminal work, *Medical Apartheid.*

36. As noted in one recent obituary, published in the *New York Times* and written in the genre of forgotten obituaries, it was evident from the start that Lacks provided scientists with some sense of possibility and futurity—even as she lay sick in Johns Hopkins. One scientist appeared on a TV science program to discuss the cells held in a bottle that he displayed to the camera: "Now let me show you a bottle in which we have grown massive quantities of cancer cells. It is quite possible that from such fundamental studies such as these that we will be able to learn a way by which cancer can be completely wiped out." The quote is attributed to Dr. George Gey. Adeel Hassan, "Henrietta Lacks: Cancer Cells Were Taken from Her Body without Permission. They Led to a Medical Revolution," *NYT Overlooked,* https://www.nytimes.com/interactive/2018/obituaries/overlooked-henrietta-lacks.html.

37. In the mid-twentieth century, the cells were sent to space and accompanied the first astronauts to the moon. They were utilized in weapons testing. Reproduced, sold, and used in research laboratories across the globe, pharmaceutical companies built multibillion-dollar empires and scientists made heroic advances and developed innumerable technologies. In 2017 German scientists published Lacks's entire genome on the internet, knowledge of which was from purchased HeLa cells. By 2018, over seventeen thousand U.S. patents were produced in connection to the HeLa cells. At the time of Skloot's book release the cells were being sold to labs, or anyone who would pay for them, for about $250 per vial.

38. "National Portrait Gallery Presents a Portrait of Henrietta Lacks, a Co-acquisition with the National Museum of African American History and Culture," National Museum of African American History and Culture, May 8, 2018, https://nmaahc.si.edu/about/news/national-portrait-gallery-presents-portrait-henrietta-lacks-co-acquisition-national.

39. Blayne Alexander, "National Portrait Gallery Opens Its Doors to Diversity with Henrietta Lacks Painting," NBC News, October 13, 2018, https://www.nbcnews.com/news/us-news/national-portrait-gallery-opens-its-doors-diversity-henrietta-lacks-painting-n919861.

40. Rebecca Skloot, *The Immortal Life of Henrietta Lacks* (New York: Broadway Paperbacks, 2010).

41. Skloot, *Immortal Life of Henrietta Lacks,* 310.

42. Skloot, 235, 302.

43. Arlene Dávila, *Latinx Art: Artists, Markets, Politics* (Durham, N.C.: Duke University Press, 2020), 20.

44. I thank Davorn Sisavath and Victor Betts for ongoing conversation about the politics of the archive, particularly for Davorn's insights on state

management of secrecy in military and government documents. See Davorn Sisavath, "The US Secret War in Laos: Constructing an Archive from Military Waste," *Radical History Review* 2019, no. 133 (2019): 103–16.

45. Sturken, *Tangled Memories*.

46. Jodi Melamed, "Racial Capitalism," *Critical Ethnic Studies* 1, no. 1 (2015): 76–78. Framing a discussion of racial capitalism, Melamed suggests that a nexus operating at the intersections of race and capitalism names the "inseparable confluence of political/economic governance with racial violence," racial violence that is naturalized by a logic of accumulation through dispossession. Melamed describes this as "the specter of race," arguing that a discourse framing race as a public threat activates legitimated state counterviolence established to protect capitalist interests in ways that would otherwise "violate social rationality." Melamed engages with *Capital* as, in part, a limitation to be used in decolonial and antiracist activist and critical ethnic studies projects: "This failure in the text of Marx brings us to the present importance of Indigenous activism and Indigenous critical theory for the task of strengthening terms of relationality that defend collective existence from racial capitalism's systematic expropriation. Neoliberalism has given us an interesting conjuncture: its rapacity for natural resources—for oil, gas, minerals, water, agricultural commodities, lumber—has required the current structure of domination to bring indigeneity into representation, because so much of the natural resources that still exist in the world are to be found on lands traditionally occupied, owned, belonging with, or stewarded by Indigenous people (up to 50 percent according to the International Forum on Globalization). This, in turn, has given Indigenous worldings a rupturous potential" (82–83).

47. Dennis Childs, *Slaves of the State: Black Incarceration from the Chain Gang to the Penitentiary* (Minneapolis: University of Minnesota Press, 2014).

48. Glen Coulthard, *Red Skin, White Masks: Rejecting the Colonial Politics of Recognition* (Minneapolis: University of Minnesota Press, 2014); TallBear, *Native American DNA*; Alondra Nelson, *Body and Soul: The Black Panther Party and the Fight against Medical Discrimination* (Minneapolis: University of Minnesota Press, 2013).

49. Michel-Rolph Trouillot, *Silencing the Past: Power and the Production of History* (New York: Random House, 2015); Lowe, *Intimacies of Four Continents*; Nelson Maldonado-Torres, *Against War: Views from the Underside of Modernity* (Durham, N.C.: Duke University Press, 2008).

50. Reddy, *Freedom with Violence*; Melamed, *Represent and Destroy*; Neda Atanasoski, *Humanitarian Violence: The U.S. Deployment of Diversity* (Minneapolis: University of Minnesota Press, 2013); Randal Williams, *The Divided World: Human Rights and Its Violence* (Minneapolis: University of Minnesota Press, 2010).

51. See recent discussions on the politics of race and techno-futurity: Neda Atanasoski and Kalindi Vora, *Surrogate Humanity: Race, Robots, and the Poli-*

tics of Technological Futures (Durham, N.C.: Duke University Press, 2019); Ruha Benjamin, *Race after Technology: Abolitionist Tools for the New Jim Code* (Cambridge: Polity, 2019); Benjamin, *Captivating Technology*; Aimee Bahng, *Migrant Futures: Decolonizing Speculation in Financial Times* (Durham, N.C.: Duke University Press, 2017).

52. Hortense J. Spillers, "Mama's Baby, Papa's Maybe," in "Culture and Countermemory: The 'American' Connection," special issue, *Diacritics* 17, no. 2 (Summer 1987): 64.

53. Melamed, *Represent and Destroy*, vi. Reading James Baldwin's "Everybody's Protest Novel" (1949) as an indicator of the shift in racial liberalism in postwar to multicultural liberalism, Melamed examines Baldwin's assessment of the protest novel in the form of *Uncle Tom's Cabin*. She suggests that it operated as the central cultural technology for transmitting racial-liberal thought at the mid-twentieth century—as the destructive normalizer of multicultural liberal systems. Melamed notes that Baldwin's understanding of abolitionist discourse as "a slight displacement" of white supremist religiosity reframed formal racisms through the form of white salvation: "For Baldwin *Uncle Tom's Cabin*, and the rationality of race and antislavery it provided, made it possible to fulfill the theological need for white salvation through abolitionism" (xii). Turning to the ways Baldwin reframed the postwar protest novel, Melamed sees it as the central cultural form invested in rationalizing violence. Melamed notes that "sociological discourses and their truth effects" had become part of "sentimental reform" and the liberal categorization of racial difference functioned as the "dominant mode for securing institutionalized conditions of knowing" (viii).

54. Hartman, *Scenes of Subjection*; Simone Browne, *Dark Matters: On the Surveillance of Blackness* (Durham, N.C.: Duke University Press, 2015).

55. Atanasoski and Vora, *Surrogate Humanity*, 6.

56. Vora, *Life Support*.

57. Atanasoski and Vora, *Surrogate Humanity*, 6.

58. TallBear, *Native American DNA*; Kim TallBear, "Caretaking Relations, Not American Dreaming," *Kalfou: A Journal of Comparative and Relational Ethnic Studies* 6, no. 1 (2019): 24.

59. See Denise Ferreira da Silva, *Toward a Global Idea of Race* (Minneapolis: University of Minnesota Press, 2007); Tiffany Willoughby-Herard, *Waste of White Skin: The Carnegie Corporation and the Racial Logic of White Vulnerability* (Berkeley: University of California Press, 2015); Ahuja, *Bioinsecurities*; Benjamin, *Race after Technology*.

60. TallBear, "Caretaking Relations, Not American Dreaming," 25. Being in relation—the spatial metaphor TallBear posits as the epistemological counterframe against liberal multiculturalism—situates other relational formations against the supposed democratic promised land of settler mythology.

61. Ferreira da Silva, *Toward a Global Idea of Race*.

62. Melamed, *Represent and Destroy*.

63. Curtis Marez, *Farm Worker Futurism: Speculative Technologies of Resistance* (Minneapolis: University of Minnesota Press, 2016). Marez theorizes what having no future in the dominant discursive imaginary means when flipped on its head through a farm worker futurism.

64. DeNeen L. Brown, "Can the 'Immortal Cells' of Henrietta Lacks Sue for Their Own Rights?," *Washington Post,* June 25, 2018, https://www.washingtonpost.com/news/retropolis/wp/2018/06/25/can-the-immortal-cells-of-henrietta-lacks-sue-for-their-own-rights/.

65. Priscilla Wald points out that Henrietta Lacks "should not have been on the ward because such a segregated space should never have existed." Priscilla Wald, "American Studies and the Politics of Life," *American Quarterly* 64, no. 2 (2012): 187–88. The question Wald ultimately pursues, posed initially in her 2011 American Studies Association presidential address and more broadly in her scholarship, is how are we to understand the unresolved, and perhaps unresolvable, tensions at the heart of medicine: "What is a cell line, and what is its relation to the human donor?" (187–88). The question I seek to examine is about that tension as it exists between definitional and transrelational concerns about ownership, property, and economies of consent.

66. Smithsonian National Museum of African American History and Culture, "National Portrait Gallery Presents a Portrait of Henrietta Lacks, a Co-acquisition with the National Museum of African American History and Culture," Museum News, May 8, 2018, https://nmaahc.si.edu/about/news/national-portrait-gallery-presents-portrait-henrietta-lacks-co-acquisition-national.

67. In the two years following the start of Donald Trump's White House, producing new structures of surveillance and policing at heightened levels and wider scales, multifaceted protests emerged. Against the Trump administration's bolstering of Immigration and Customs Enforcement, large-scale marches moved through the capital. Organized protests challenging threats to reproductive rights and ruptures around the face-off between an American Indian activist and MAGA-hat-wearing teenagers highlighted the ongoing resistance forming alongside the theorizing of Black Lives Matter movements and critiques.

68. As I write this Introduction, Native and Indigenous protectors and allies protest Donald Trump's decision to hold a politically symbolic photo op in the sacred lands of the Black Hills. Trump's decision to further politicize state memory and white nationalism during Covid-19 was clearly designed to challenge tribal sovereignty, as Cheyenne River, Oglala, and Rosebud Sioux Tribes and leaders demand it. See "Trump Must Respect Sovereignty When He Visits Mt. Rushmore on July 3," *Indian Country Today,* July 2, 2020, https://indiancountrytoday.com/opinion/trump-must-respect-sovereignty-when-he-visits-mt-rushmore-on-july-3-92zYVI3flkm7CVJura3wpQ.

69. "UC San Diego Recognizes Black History Month with Events Cel-

ebrating Achievements of African-American Women," UC San Diego Today, January 31, 2012, https://today.ucsd.edu/story/campus_recognizes_black_his tory_month_with_events_celebrating_achievements.

70. Ruha Benjamin, "Introduction: Discriminatory Design, Liberating Imag- ination," in *Captivating Technology: Race, Carceral Technoscience, and Libera- tory Imagination in Everyday Life*, ed. Ruha Benjamin, 1–14 (Durham, N.C.: Duke University Press, 2019).

71. See Britt Rusert, "Naturalizing Coercion: The Tuskegee Experiments and the Laboratory Life of the Plantation," in *Captivating Technology: Race, Carceral Technoscience, and Liberatory Imagination in Everyday Life*, ed. Ruha Benjamin, 25–49 (Durham, N.C.: Duke University Press, 2019); Allen M. Hornblum, *Acres of Skin: Human Experiments at Holmesburg Prison* (London: Routledge, 1999); James H. Jones, *Bad Blood: The Tuskegee Syphilis Experiment* (New York: Free Press, 1993); Washington, *Medical Apartheid*.

72. Nelson, *Body and Soul*, xi. Nelson continues: "Activists, too, were con- versant in the political rhetoric of the health crisis. In diametric contrast with the Nixon administration and healthcare lobbyists who were commit- ted to the continued commodification of medical care, health radicals—a coterie that included the Black Panther Party, health workers such as the MCHR and the Student Health Organization (SHO), and the New Left- oriented Health Policy Advisory Center (or Health/PAC)—understood the most acute aspect of the crisis to be the proliferation of a capitalist medical system that produced and exacerbated inequality. The Chicago Black Panther Party minister of health Ronald 'Doc' Satchel's complaint in the pages of the *Black Panther* [newsletter] that 'the medical profession within this capital- ist society . . . is composed generally of people working for their own benefit and advancement rather than the humane aspects of medical care' typified this activist argument. The health Left often parted ways with liberal reform- ers, such as Senator Kennedy, who believed that mainstream medicine could be made more equitable. For these radicals, a for-profit healthcare system was fundamentally and inherently flawed. Accordingly, they took no suc- cor in the proliferation of the medical-industrial complex—even in a liberal guise" (14).

73. Ferreira da Silva, *Toward a Global Idea of Race*, xxxv.

74. Lowe, *Intimacies of Four Continents*, 2–3.

75. Lowe, "History Hesitant," 85.

76. Lowe, 85.

77. I gratefully note Salar Mameni, Chien-ting Lin, and Joo Ok Kim for the ongoing dialogue on this question of recovery. Thanks to Salar for the push to explore connections between "recovery" of the archive and *recovery* as a medi- calized term with social, cultural, and political valences.

78. Jonathan Kamakawiwoʻole Osorio, *Dismembering Lāhui: A History of the Hawaiian Nation to 1887* (Honolulu: University of Hawaiʻi Press, 2002).

79. David A. Chang, *The World and All the Things upon It: Native Hawaiian Geographies of Exploration* (Minneapolis: University of Minnesota Press, 2016), viii.

80. Melamed, *Represent and Destroy*, xiii–xiv; Atanasoski, *Humanitarian Violence*, 9; Grace Kyungwon Hong and Roderick A. Ferguson, *Strange Affinities: The Gender and Sexual Politics of Comparative Racialization* (Durham, N.C.: Duke University Press, 2011); Grace Kyungwon Hong, *Death beyond Disavowal: The Impossible Politics of Difference* (Minneapolis: University of Minnesota Press, 2015); Reddy, *Freedom with Violence*.

81. See Rosaura Sánchez and Beatrice Pita, *Spatial and Discursive Violence in the U.S. Southwest* (Durham, N.C.: Duke University Press, 2021).

82. Melamed, *Represent and Destroy*, 13; Scott Richard Lyons, *X-Marks: Native Signatures of Assent* (Minneapolis: University of Minnesota Press, 2010).

83. Saidiya Hartman, "The Death Toll," in *The Quarantine Files: Thinkers in Self-Isolation*, ed. Brad Evans (Los Angeles: Los Angeles Review of Books, 2020), https://lareviewofbooks.org/article/quarantine-files-thinkers -self-isolation/#_ftn15.

1. Medical Violence, Archival Fictions

1. Lisa Lowe, *The Intimacies of Four Continents* (Durham, N.C.: Duke University Press, 2015), 2–3.

2. Anonymous, "The Contagious Nature of Leprosy," *British Medical Journal* 1 (1890): 917–18.

3. "King vs. Keanu: Opinions of Judd C. J. on Motion for New Trial," July 18, 1884, Box 1052: Criminal, Folder 002: Criminal Case Files of the First Circuit Court, Hawai'i State Archives.

4. Chief Justice Albert Francis Judd (1838–1900), son of physician Gerrit P. Judd (1803–1873) and Laura Fish Judd (1804–1872), was a central colonial figure in nineteenth century Hawai'i. The Judd family lineage ties to Thomas Hastings, puritan colonist of the Massachusetts Bay Colony who arrived from East Anglia in 1634. Judd's father was part of one of the earliest waves of missionaries (the American Board of Commissioners for Foreign Missions) in Hawai'i, the author of the first medical publications translated into the Hawaiian language, a member of the cabinet of King Kamehameha III, and the owner of the Kualoa Ranch, which consists of over four thousand acres of land purchased throughout the nineteenth century (currently owned by his descendants). As Chief Justice, Albert Francis Judd was significant in ushering in the U.S. annexation (1898) and territorial government.

5. "King vs. Keanu." For an early discussion of the case proceedings within the context of medical history, see Arthur Albert St. M. Mouritz, *The Path of the Destroyer: A History of Leprosy in the Hawaiian Islands and Thirty Years Research into the Means by Which It Has Been Spread* (Honolulu: Honolulu Star-Bulletin, 1916), 153; Kerri A. Inglis, *Ma'i Lepera: A History of Leprosy in Nineteenth-Century Hawai'i* (Honolulu: University of Hawai'i Press, 2013).

6. "The Kohala Murder Case," *Pacific Commercial Advertiser* (Honolulu), July 22, 1884, found in Library of Congress, Chronicling America: Historic American Newspapers, http://chroniclingamerica.loc.gov/lccn/sn82015418/1884-07 -22/ed-1/seq-15/.

7. Wright, "The Inoculability of Leprosy," *British Medical Journal* 2 (1888), 1359.

8. Privy Council. "Reign of Kalakaua. King," August 13, 1884, Vol. 14; page 131, Hawai'i State Archives.

9. O. A. Bushnell, "Dr. Edward Arning, the First Microbiologist in Hawaii," *Hawaiian Journal of History* 1 (1967): 3; Nicholas Turse, "Experimental Dreams, Ethical Nightmares: Leprosy, Isolation, and Human Experimentation in Nineteenth-Century Hawaii," in *Imagining Our Americas: Toward a Transnational Frame,* ed. Sandhya Shukla and Heidi Tinsman (Durham, N.C.: Duke University Press, 2007), 138.

10. Heráclides César de Souza Araújo, from his "A lepra e as organizações anti-leprosas do Brasil em 1936: 2.- Estado do Pará—Organizações anti-leprosas: Lazaropolis do Prata." Mem. Inst. Osw. Cruz, 1937:32 (1), quoted in Jaime L. Benchimol and Magali Romero Sá, "Adolpho Lutz and the Controversies over Leprosy," in *Adolpho Lutz-Hanseníase-v. 1, Livro 2* (Editora Fiocruz, 2004), 195. Souza Araújo (1886–1962) was a Brazilian scientist and scientific biographer who was well known and highly respected for his twentieth-century research on containing and treating Hansen's disease.

11. The significance of the 1865 Act to Prevent the Spread of Leprosy and the settlement on Kalaupapa, Moloka'i, have been discussed widely and continue to be a flashpoint for critical scholarship. For this discussion, see Pennie Moblo, "Defamation by Disease: Leprosy, Myth, and Ideology in Nineteenth-Century Hawai'i" (PhD diss., University of Hawai'i, 1996); Inglis, *Ma'i Lepera*; Michelle T. Moran, *Colonizing Leprosy: Imperialism and the Politics of Public Health in the United States* (Chapel Hill: University of North Carolina Press, 2007); Noenoe K. Silva, *Aloha Betrayed: Native Hawaiian Resistance to American Colonialism* (Durham, N.C.: Duke University Press, 2004); Neel Ahuja, *Bioinsecurities: Disease Interventions, Empire, and the Government of Species* (Durham, N.C.: Duke University Press, 2016), 29–70.

12. For an expansive analysis of nineteenth-century colonial and imperial politics in Hawai'i, see Jonathan Kay Kamakawiwo'ole Osorio, *Dismembering Lāhui: A History of the Hawaiian Nation to 1887* (Honolulu: University of Hawai'i Press, 2002).

13. Inglis, *Ma'i Lepera,* 1.

14. Inglis, 17–77. Inglis specifically discusses the criminal case of prisoner-patient Native Hawaiian Keanu, the focus of this chapter. Notable analysis of the significance of this case to colonial medicine could be said to begin with Mouritz's *Path of the Destroyer,* discussed in detail in Ahuja, *Bioinsecurities,* 29–70. See also O. A. Bushnell, *The Gifts of Civilization: Germs and Genocide in Hawai'i* (Honolulu: University of Hawai'i Press, 1993). Bushnell, whose fiction is

discussed in this chapter, presents a critical analysis of colonial medicine and imperial violence across the Pacific Islands.

15. Act to Prevent the Spread of Leprosy, 1865 (quote from full document in English in Inglis, *Maʻi Lepera*, Appendix B, 203–5). "Section 3. The Board of Health or its agents, are authorized and empowered to cause to be isolated and confined, in some place or places for the purpose provided, all leprous patients who shall be deemed capable of spreading the disease of Leprosy; and it shall be the duty of every Police and District Justice, when properly applied to that purpose by the Board of Health, or its authorized agents, to cause to be arrested and delivered to the Board of Health or its agents, any person alleged to be a leper, within the jurisdiction of such Police or District Justice; and it shall be the duty of the Marshal of the Hawaiian Islands and his Deputies, and of the Police Officers, to assist in securing the conveyance of any person so arrested, to such place as the Board of Health or its agents may direct, in order that such person may be subjected to medical inspection, and thereafter to assist in removing such a person to a place of treatment, or isolation, if so required by the agents of the Board of Health."

16. Ahuja, *Bioinsecurities*, 29–70. In addition to drawing out the global connections in Ahuja's study, regarding specifically transitory movements of medical knowledge in colonial contexts, the focus on how this situates people under criminalizing logics is key to how I am reading the medical archive. "In addition to subjecting Hawaiian 'leprosy suspects' to enforced policing screenings for skin lesions and other symptoms, those infected were criminalized and termed alternatively and ambiguously in early Board of Health documents as 'prisoners' and 'patients'" (33). See also Moran, *Colonizing Leprosy*.

17. J. Kēhaulani Kauanui, *Hawaiian Blood: Colonialism and the Politics of Sovereignty and Indigeneity* (Durham, N.C.: Duke University Press, 2008); Glen Sean Coulthard, *Red Skin, White Masks: Rejecting the Colonial Politics of Recognition* (Minneapolis: University of Minnesota Press, 2014); Aileen Moreton-Robinson, *The White Possessive: Property, Power, and Indigenous Sovereignty* (Minneapolis: University of Minnesota Press, 2015).

18. Bushnell, "Dr. Edward Arning," 3. In the negotiations for this stipend, Bushnell notes: "Arning's sponsors were two of Germany's most prestigious scientists: Dr. Rudolf Virchow, the foremost pathologist of his time, and Dr. Emil du Bois-Reymond, an eminent physiologist." Reprints of Dr. Arning's photography collection can be found in the Eduard Arning Photograph Collection: 1883–1886 at the Hawaiian Historical Society Library.

19. Bushnell, "Dr. Edward Arning," 4.

20. Lowe, *Intimacies of Four Continents*; Danika Medak-Saltzman, "Transnational Indigenous Exchange: Rethinking Global Interactions of Indigenous Peoples at the 1904 St. Louis Exposition," *American Quarterly* 62, no. 3 (2010): 591. On reframing the question of coloniality, power, history, and the archive, see also Silva, *Aloha Betrayed*; Kamanamaikalani Beamer, *No Mākou ka Mana:*

Liberating the Nation (Honolulu: Kamehameha Publishing, 2015). Glen Sean Coulthard defines a settler-colonial relationship as "one characterized by a particular form of domination; that is, it is a relationship where power—in this case, interrelated discursive and non-discursive facets of economic, gendered, racial, and state power—has been structured into a relatively secure or sedimented set of hierarchical social relations that continue to facilitate the dispossession of Indigenous peoples of their lands and self-determining authority." Coulthard, *Red Skin, White Masks*, 6–7.

21. See H. P. Wright, *Statutes of the Hospital of the Holy Virgin Mary of Siena, AD 1305, Tr. by H. P. Wright* (1880), xv.; *Leprosy and Segregation* (London: Parker and Co., 1885); "Leprosy: An Imperial Danger," *American Journal of the Medical Sciences* 98, no. 6 (1889); "The Spread of Leprosy," *British Medical Journal* (1889). Wright published extensively in the 1880s and 1890s promoting his view that leprosy in the colonies posed an imminent threat to European nations.

22. See O. A. Bushnell, *Molokai: A Novel* (Honolulu: University of Hawai'i Press, 1975).

23. For a broader context of imperial medicine and the insights gained from colonial practice, as well as resistance to them, see Warwick Anderson, *Colonial Pathologies: American Tropical Medicine, Race, and Hygiene in the Philippines* (Durham, N.C.: Duke University Press, 2006); Inglis, *Ma'i Lepera*.

24. Beaven Rake, "Leprosy and Vaccination," *British Medical Journal* 2 (1887): 443.

25. John Tayman, *The Colony: The Harrowing True Story of the Exiles of Molokai* (New York: Scribner, 2007), 147.

26. Rake, "Leprosy and Vaccination," 443.

27. "King vs. Keanu: Motion to Change Place of Trial," May 8, 1884, Box 1052: Criminal, Folder 002: Criminal Case Files of the First Circuit Court, Hawai'i State Archives.

28. Moreton-Robinson, *White Possessive*, xxiv; Cheryl Harris, "Whiteness as Property," *Harvard Law Review* 106 (1992): 1,707; Maile Renee Arvin, "Pacifically Possessed: Scientific Production and Native Hawaiian Critique of the 'Almost White' Polynesian Race" (PhD diss., University of California, San Diego, 2013).

29. Rake, "Leprosy and Vaccination," 433; Jonathan Hutchinson, "Remarks on Some Facts Illustrating the Early Stages of Leprosy," *British Medical Journal* 1 (1890): 529–31; Bushnell, "Dr. Edward Arning," 3; Mouritz, *Path of the Destroyer*, 152.

30. Lowe locates such narrative processes within what she terms the archives of liberalism. Lowe asserts that in examining state archives produced by such historical events, we can better interrogate "the ways in which the archive that mediates the imperatives of the state subsumes colonial violence within narratives of modern reason and progress." To critically examine the colonial archive at the center of "forcible encounters, removals, and entanglements

[that have been] omitted in liberal accounts of abolition, emancipation, and independence," Lowe argues for other ways of reading that resist the processes through which "the forgetting of violent encounter is naturalized, both by the archive, and in the subsequent narrative histories." Lowe, *Intimacies of Four Continents,* 2–3.

31. Lowe, 3.

32. For two discussions on cultural fantasies of the Pacific, see Paul Lyons, *American Pacificism: Oceania in the U.S. Imagination* (New York: Routledge, 2006) and Rob Wilson, *Reimagining the American Pacific: From South Pacific to Bamboo Ridge and Beyond* (Durham, N.C.: Duke University Press, 2000). In another context, Rona Tamiko Halualani locates such narrative processes in longer historical narratives of colonization—a phenomenon she calls "abstract nativism." Rona Tamiko Halualani, *In the Name of Hawaiians: Native Identities and Cultural Politics* (Minneapolis: University of Minnesota Press, 2002), 6.

33. Noenoe K. Silva describes one of "the most persistent and pernicious myths of Hawaiian history" as "the Kanaka Maoli (Native Hawaiians) passively accept[ing] the erosion of their culture and loss of their nation." Silva's study refutes the myth through documentation and study of "the many forms of resistance by the Kanaka Maoli to political, economic, linguistic, and cultural oppression, beginning with the arrival of Captain Cook until the struggle over the 'annexation,' that is, the military occupation of Hawai'i by the United States in 1898." Silva, *Aloha Betrayed,* 1.

34. Moreton-Robinson, *White Possessive,* 50.

35. Wright, "Inoculability of Leprosy," 1,359.

36. For a discussion of biopower and state racism, see Michel Foucault, *"Society Must Be Defended": Lectures at the College de France, 1975–1976* (New York: Picador, 2003), 239–64. For an interrogation and further development of Foucault's concept of biopower, see Achille Mbembe, "Necropolitics," *Public Culture* 15, no. 1 (2003): 11–40.

37. Wright, "Inoculability of Leprosy," 1,359.

38. In Moreton-Robinson's framing, such subject formations emerged directly out of Indigenous dispossession: "Most historians mark 1492 as the year when imperialism began to construct the old world order by taking possession of other people, their lands and resources. The possessive nature of this enterprise informed the development of a racial stratification process on a global scale that became solidified in modernity. Taking possession of Indigenous people's lands was a quintessential act of colonization and was tied to the tradition from the Enlightenment to modernity, which precipitated the emergence of a new subject into history within Europe." Moreton-Robinson, *White Possessive,* 49.

39. Lowe, *Intimacies of Four Continents,* 2.

40. Jodi Byrd, *The Transit of Empire: Indigenous Critiques of Colonialism* (Minneapolis: University of Minnesota Press, 2011); Rosaura Sánchez and Bea-

trice Pita, *Spatial and Discursive Violence in the U.S. Southwest* (Durham, N.C.: Duke University Press, 2021).

41. Scott Richard Lyons, *X-Marks: Native Signatures of Assent* (Minneapolis: University of Minnesota Press, 2010), 1.

42. Jonathan Kay Kamakawiwoʻole Osorio argues that Hawaiian sovereignty was subjected to processes of dismemberment, not only through direct and physical seizing of lands "but through a slow, insinuating invasion of people, ideas, and institutions." Osorio, *Dismembering Lāhui*, 3. Reverend Richard Armstrong and his family, sent to the Marquesas Islands and Hawaiʻi in the 1830s by the American Board of Commissioners for Foreign Missions (ABCFM), wrote often about the need to "teach the young natives" civilized behavior because, for Hawaiians, "to lie and steal seemed as natural as to breathe." Armstrong described Hawaiians as "very repulsive in their personal habits and immoral in the extreme. . . . Week after week passes and we see none but naked, filthy, wicked heathen with souls as dark as the tabernacles which they inhabit" (99). Armstrong, in a policy recommendation in 1846 to the Hawaiian king's minister of foreign relations, Robert C. Wyllie, states: "I think an effort should be made to connect some sort of manual labor, especially agriculture, with all the schools. . . . Early habits of industry will supply their wants, make their homes comfortable and remove the temptation to wander about and commit crime in order to get money or fine dress" (103). Osorio notes that missionary thought was one of the central factors for the successful and thorough colonization of nineteenth-century Hawaiʻi, where the focus was not only on "a slow, insinuating invasion of people, ideas, and institutions" but also articulating a Hawaiian subject that possessed individual rights and claims to both personhood and property (3). Religious leaders in Hawaiʻi in the early and mid-nineteenth century were explicit about this point, as Hiram Bingham, leader of the ABCFM, wrote in his memoirs that the ultimate goal was "to introduce and extend among them the more useful art and usages of civilized and Christianized society, and to fill the habitable parts of those important islands with schools and churches, fruitful fields and pleasant dwellings" (19).

43. Luana Ross, *Inventing the Savage: The Social Construction of Native American Criminality* (Austin: University of Texas Press, 1998), 5.

44. Ross addresses histories of American Indians in Montana. The framework developed in Ross's work connects to the lack of recognition of self-determination, eliding, in the official narratives, Native sovereignty and subjectivity as autonomous, complex, and historically situated and racialized.

45. Giorgio Agamben, *Homo Sacer: Sovereign Power and Bare Life*, trans. Daniel Heller-Roazen (Stanford, Calif.: Stanford University Press, 1998), 156. Giorgio Agamben calls attention to the significance of medical state-sanctioned violence, for example, noting that it is hardly an exceptional characteristic but rather an indication of the legitimacy produced and expressed by these institutions. He notes the use of the figure of Keanu as justification for Nazi human

experimentation at Dachau. Pointing to the ethical and logical hoops necessary to jump through when utilizing prisoner consent, Agamben details a long history of medicine benefiting from incarcerated bodies: "What is . . . disquieting is the fact (which is unequivocally shown by the scientific literature put forward by the defense and confirmed by the expert witnesses appointed by the court) that experiments on prisoners and persons sentenced to death had been performed several times and on a large scale in our century, in particular in the United States (the very country from which most of the Nuremberg judges came). Thus in the 1920s, 800 people held in United States prisons were infected with malaria plasmodia in an attempt to find an antidote to paludism. There were also the experiments—widely held to be exemplary in the scientific literature on pellagra—conducted by Goldberg on twelve prisoners sentenced to death, who were promised the remission of their penalty if they survived experimentation. Outside the United States, the first experiments with cultures of the beriberi bacillus were conducted by R. P. Strong in Manila on persons sentenced to death (the records of the experiment do not mention whether participation in the experiment was voluntary). In addition, the defense cited the case of Keanu (Hawaii), who was infected with leprosy in order to be promised pardon, and who died following the experiment" (90).

46. Anonymous, "The Case of Keanu," *New Orleans Medical and Surgical Journal* 43 (1890): 87.

47. Wright, "Inoculability of Leprosy," 1,359.

48. Tayman, *Colony,* 147.

49. See the long history of racial medical violence in Harriet A. Washington, *Medical Apartheid: The Dark History of Medical Experimentation on Black Americans from Colonial Times to the Present* (New York: Doubleday, 2006).

50. Anonymous, "Contagious Nature of Leprosy," 917.

51. Arning's collections are kept in Hawai'i and Berlin, Germany. The photo of Keanu I examined is housed at the Hawaiian Historical Society Library's Eduard Arning Photograph Collection: 1883–1886.

52. Tony Gould, *A Disease Apart: Leprosy in the Modern World* (New York: St. Martin's Press, 2005), 83.

53. Anonymous, "Contagious Nature of Leprosy," 918.

54. Anonymous, 918.

55. Anonymous, "Shall We Annex Leprosy? By a Hawaiian Government School Teacher," *Cosmopolitan: A Monthly Illustrated Magazine,* no. 24, 1897, 557–61. Reference to Keanu and Arning appeared in this widely circulated 1898 *Cosmopolitan* essay. The anonymous author contributed to antiannexation debates at their peak, as the United States government was maneuvering to overthrow the Kingdom of Hawai'i in 1898. The author asserts the racist discourse that the annexation would provide an entryway for the east to infect the United States through racially mixing as well as through contagious diseases. Arning and Keanu are discussed, though not named: "Some eminent scientists

in Honolulu have been experimenting. They tried the virus on a man who was condemned to be hanged and he was sent to Molokai as a leper" (560).

56. Wright, "Inoculability of Leprosy," 1,359.

57. Anthony Bogues, *Empire of Liberty: Power, Desire, and Freedom* (Lebanon, N.H.: University Press of New England, 2010), 18–19.

58. Bogues, *Empire of Liberty,* 19.

59. Wright, "Inoculability of Leprosy," 1,359.

60. Wright, 1,359.

61. For Arning's full analysis of the experiments and, more broadly, his evaluation of Hansen's disease in Hawai'i, see the official report he submitted to the Board of Health. "Report of Edward Arning, M.D., on Leprosy, November 14th 1885," Series 334–35, Folder "Dr. Edward Arning: 1883–1888," Board of Health, Hansen's Disease, Hawai'i State Archives.

62. Lowe, *Intimacies of Four Continents,* 4.

63. Bushnell, *Molokai,* 68.

64. Bushnell, 67.

65. Bushnell, 49.

66. For discussions on fantasy and the national U.S. imaginary, see Jason Berger, *Antebellum at Sea: Maritime Fantasies in Nineteenth-Century America* (Minneapolis: University of Minnesota Press, 2012); Hester Blum, *The View from the Masthead: Maritime Imagination and Antebellum American Sea Narratives* (Chapel Hill: University of North Carolina Press, 2008); Ward Churchill, *Fantasies of the Master Race: Literature, Cinema, and Colonization of American Indians* (San Francisco: City Lights Books, 1992); Lyons, *American Pacificism*; Wilson, *Reimagining the American Pacific.* Drawing on Edward Said's *Orientalism,* Paul Lyons argues that Herman Melville's travel writing looms large in Western ideologies, suggesting that his cultural work provides a script of American Pacificism. Jason Berger notes that such fantasies have "significant political import in this era, for they emerge (or reemerge) to organize, condition, and respond to experiences in which social, political, and economic antagonisms often occurred or came to a head." Berger, *Antebellum at Sea,* 4. The "problem of the sea" in cultural production, Berger suggests, is perpetually framed not by contact between colonial and colonized subjects so much as by the "limitations" that writers such as Melville face when attempting to represent ocean and island life as a "coherent cultural and imaginative space." Scholars have sought to explore the implications of fantasy and the maritime imaginary within the context of U.S. national formations. Such representations reveal not only a cultural production of limited knowledge and exposure but also an extension of the discursive manifestation of subjects exceeding legal spheres in colonial spaces. Elizabeth Maddock Dillon argues for a more explicit return to the cultural as a site of contestation, noting that "representation (and the political power attached to representation)" should be understood in terms of the "arenas of cultural contestation and meaning making that have political

force and value." Elizabeth Maddock Dillon, *New World Drama: The Performative Commons in the Atlantic World, 1649–1849* (Durham, N.C.: Duke University Press, 2014), 9. As markers of contestation, the shape of cultural representation reflects a continuous engagement by cultural producers and consumers alike, and I would add that it signifies the location of a site of tension around those represented.

  67. Brian Roberts and Michelle Stephens, introduction to *Archipelagic American Studies*, ed. Brian Roberts and Michelle Stephens (Durham, N.C.: Duke University Press, 2014), 3. Roberts and Stephens argue for an "archipelagic turn" in American studies and to develop analytics that account for representation of archipelagoes across the globe that does not relegate island space and peoples to a continentally determined understanding of social and cultural logics of modernity. Also see their special issue, an early version of the above edited volume: Brian Roberts and Michelle Stephens, "Archipelagic American Studies and the Caribbean," *Journal of Transnational American Studies* 5, no. 1 (2013): 1–20. In the introduction to that special issue, they note: "[Americanist] scholars . . . have only deployed the term insular according to what is a widely accepted usage, namely to describe a state of being 'cut off from intercourse with other nations, isolated; self-contained; narrow or prejudiced in feelings, ideas, or manners.' But it is important to trace and remark on the entrenched epistemic violence resulting from and perpetuated by a continentally oriented (neo)colonial modernity that has looked toward the island's defining geoformal attribute and ascribed to it this derogatory second meaning, which ineluctably links island-space (and by extension island peoples) to an anti-cosmopolitan mentality" (3).

  68. Bushnell, "Dr. Edward Arning," 9.

  69. Bushnell, *Gifts of Civilization.*

  70. Bushnell, "Dr. Edward Arning," 9.

  71. Stephen Sumida, *And the View from the Shore: Literary Traditions of Hawai'i* (Seattle: University of Washington Press, 1991), 192.

  72. Paul Lyons, "Wayne Kaumualii Westlake, Richard Hamasaki, and the Afterlives of (Native/Non-Native) Collaboration against Empire in Hawai'i," *Anglistica* 14, no. 2 (2010): 81. On localism in Hawai'i, statehood and cultural nationalisms, and tensions surrounding the location and definitions of literary conventions and aesthetics, Lyons notes: "The fault lines within such 'localism,' in its literary form, became evident in the mid-1980s, and were debated through the 1990s, breaking around the question of whether Hawai'i was to be thought of as affectively part of 'America'—as region, 'local' movement, or sub-nation within it, for which 'Bamboo Ridge' (the focal point of much of the debate about the politics of 'local' literature, despite, or because, its editors take a generally apolitical stance toward literature) might figure as sign—or taken to be an occupied/colonized place, whose subjects might form alliances internally, articulating their politics with indigenous claims, in support of the

principle of sovereignty, and externally, in relation to decolonizing movements in the Pacific and elsewhere. To dissident creative writer/artists in Hawai'i, the call of the U.S. state to a participatory citizenship built on Hawaiian displacement or legal assimilation inspires no affective loyalty."

73. Dean Itsuji Saranillio, *Unsustainable Empire: Alternative Histories of Hawai'i* (Durham, N.C.: Duke University Press, 2018), xii.

74. In *And the View from the Shore*'s "Hawaii's Local Literary Tradition," Sumida notes that Bushnell was a medical historian at the University of Hawai'i, an established writer of historical fiction about Hawai'i, and a "Hawai'i-born, third-generation descendant of a mix of European immigrants to Hawai'i including Portuguese and Norwegians," allowing Bushnell to grow up "learning to read the pulse of the land and its people" (164). Accordingly, Sumida suggests that Bushnell set out to challenge "local" Hawaiian writers to do more to represent Hawai'i's ethnic voice, counternarratives to those written by "outsiders" (277).

75. Sumida's reflections on the famous conference Story Talk: Words Bind, Words Set Free were published in 1986 in *The Best of Bamboo Ridge: The Hawaii Writers' Quarterly,* ed. Eric Chock and Darrell H. Y. Lum (Honolulu: Bamboo Ridge Press, 1986), 302–21. Sumida addresses an enduring belief that "Hawaii's local people have been stereotyped as being silent or quiet, not merely reticent but deficient in verbal skills and therefore incapable of creating literature of any merit, much less a literary tradition." Sumida, *And the View from the Shore,* 277. Sumida is responding, in part, to Bushnell's critique of ethnic Hawaiian writers (specifically Asian American writers of Hawai'i)—comments Bushnell presented as the opening keynote address to the 1978 Talk Story: Our Voices in Literature and Song—Hawaii's Ethnic American Writers' Conference.

76. See reference to Talk Story: Our Voices in Literature and Song—Hawaii's Ethnic American Writers' Conference, quoted in Sumida, *And the View from the Shore,* 239.

77. Saranillio discusses the significance of Michener as the cultural side of the political discourse of pro-statehood, describing Hawai'i as an extension of historical arguments underpinning the state movement as "racial narratives." Saranillio states: "This played out in [Kathleen Dickenson Mellen's] public criticism and arguments with Michener's first epic novel titled *Hawaii,* written as a manifesto of the statehood movement and published in 1959 only a few months after statehood was achieved. Michener's arguments gained legitimacy by tying themselves to the scholarship of the University of Hawai'i Department of Sociology. By 1978, Michener's *Hawaii* had sold five million copies." Saranillio, *Unsustainable Empire,* 160.

78. Sumida, *And the View from the Shore,* 302. Sumida traces Bushnell's statements to Michener and his widely read novel *Hawaii,* which implied that there was no Asian American literary voice in Hawai'i. Sumida states: "In 1959, Hawaii gained U.S. statehood, having been a territory since annexation in 1898.

Not by mere coincidence, in 1959 two books important to Hawaii's literature were published. . . . One is James A. Michener's novel, *Hawaii.* . . . Michener's came to be known as *the* novel of Hawaii. . . . Michener and scholar A. Grove Day counter these charges with the obvious disclaimer that the novel is, after all, fiction. But there has also been another dissatisfaction with the novel among certain people in Hawaii: that the novel considered to be *the* novel of Hawaii has been written by an outsider. Why did no one born and raised in Hawaii, someone steeped in the ways and the knowledge of Hawaii's cultures and history, write the novel? Why did no one among each of the major ethnic groups of whom Michener writes tell his or her people's story from the inside out? The dissatisfaction was also that somehow we in Hawaii had been robbed, and now it was too late to overtake the thief. And it was our own fault—somehow" (302–3).

79.   Scholars and activists chart how this political maneuver came to be; see Haunani-Kay Trask, *From a Native Daughter: Colonialism and Sovereignty in Hawai'i* (Honolulu: University of Hawai'i Press, 1999), 30, 235; J. Kēhaulani Kauanui, "Colonialism in Equality: Hawaiian Sovereignty and the Question of U.S. Civil Rights," *South Atlantic Quarterly* 107, no. 4 (Fall 2008): 643; Adria Imada, *Aloha America: Hula Circuits through the U.S. Empire* (Durham, N.C.: Duke University Press, 2012), 274. Adria Imada notes that Congress "passed a bill making the territory the fiftieth state of the union and Hawai'i's population approved statehood via plebiscite. However, this plebiscite offered only two choices on the ballot: statehood or continued territorial status. Furthermore, military personnel and non-Hawaiians who outnumbered Kanaka Maoli were allowed to vote." As late as the 1880s, "hula was resurrected and enshrined by the Hawaiian monarchy as an anti-imperial, state-sponsored form of national revival in defiance of haole missionary settlers." Imada, *Aloha America,* 11. Similarly, in *Aloha Betrayed: Native Hawaiian Resistance to American Colonialism,* Noenoe K. Silva unsettles what she and others call the enduring myths of Hawai'i not only by employing Foucault's frameworks of "madness, illness, death, crime, sexuality, and so forth" but also by foregrounding the study of colonialism in the Pacific Islands (6). Silva disrupts the "persistent and pernicious myths" portraying Hawaiian history and culture as passively accepting the "erosion of their culture and the loss of their nation," and her archival research reveals how Native residents regularly resisted colonialism. Silva notes, as one example, the Kalaupapa settlement on Moloka'i in the late nineteenth century. Residents, despite being quarantined as "lepers" and imprisoned on the peninsula, protested before and after the U.S. annexation of Hawai'i, and leaders in the Kalaupapa community "not only gathered signatures on the protest petitions, but earlier had organized a full day of activities to commemorate the queen's birthday on September 2" (149–50). Bushnell's statements at the 1978 Talk Story conference reflect conversations extending from early moments of colonialism to cultural and political contexts around the question of Hawaiian cultural renaissance

and sovereignty movements in the twentieth century. In the 1980s, not long
after the Talk Story conference, Haunani-Kay Trask published on the ways in
which Native Hawaiian interests were elided not only by North American and
European colonial legacies but also by growing economic pressures from Asia,
directly affecting Hawai'i and the Pacific Islands more broadly. Trask writes
on the impact of Japanese tourism on Native Hawaiians as it moves "into the
Pacific with aggressive economic penetration as investors and as tourists in
Vanuatu, Tahiti, Micronesia, Fiji, Sāmoa, and elsewhere." The shift in global
influences on the Pacific Islands, Trask notes, is felt most as travel increases
through tourism: "In Hawai'i, Japanese firms have purchased over nine billion
dollars worth of real estate since the 1970s." See Haunani-Kay Trask, "Apolo-
gies," in *Asian Settler Colonialism: From Local Governance to the Habits of Everyday Life in Hawai'i,* ed. Candace Fujikane and Jonathan Y. Okamura (Honolulu:
University of Hawai'i Press, 2008): 50. In the introduction to *Asian Settler Colonialism,* Candace Fujikane writes: "Read in the context of Hawaiian scholarship on U.S. colonialism . . . ethnic histories written about Asians in Hawai'i
demonstrate an investment in the ideal of American democracy that is ideo-
logically at odds with indigenous critiques of U.S. colonialism. Although these
historical accounts often recognize that Hawaiians have a unique political status as indigenous peoples, they do not address the roles of Asians in an American colonial system. Instead, they recount Asian histories of oppression and
resistance in Hawai'i, erecting a multicultural ethnic studies framework that
ends up reproducing the colonial claims made in white settler historiography.
In their focus on racism, discrimination, and the exclusion of Asians from full
participation in an American democracy, such studies tell the story of Asians'
civil rights struggles as one of nation building in order to legitimate Asians'
claims to a place for themselves in Hawai'i." Candance Fujikane, introduction
to *Asian Settler Colonialism: From Local Governance to the Habits of Everyday
Life in Hawai'i,* ed. Candace Fujikane and Jonathan Y. Okamura (Honolulu: University of Hawai'i Press, 2008), 2. Also see Wilson, *Reimagining the American
Pacific*; Edward Beechert, *Working in Hawaii: A Labor History* (Honolulu: University of Hawai'i Press, 1985); Moon-Kie Jung, *Reworking Race: The Making of
Hawaii's Interracial Labor Movement* (New York: University of Columbia Press,
1985); Gary Okihiro, *Cane Fires: The Anti-Japanese Movement in Hawaii, 1865–
1945* (Philadelphia: Temple University Press, 1991); Gary Okihiro, *Pineapple
Culture: A History of the Tropical and Temperate Zones* (Berkeley: University of
California Press, 2009); Judy Rohrer, *Haoles in Hawai'i: Race and Ethnicity in
Hawai'i* (Honolulu: University of Hawai'i Press, 2010); Ronald Takaki, *Pau Hana:
Plantation Life and Labor in Hawaii, 1835–1920* (Honolulu: University of Hawai'i
Press, 1983).

   80. See Bushnell's other novels: *Ka'a'awa: A Novel about Hawaii in the 1850s*
(Honolulu: University of Hawai'i Press, 1972), which fictionalizes the impact
of smallpox on O'ahu in the 1850s; *Stone of Kannon* (Honolulu: Friends of the

Library of Hawaii, 1979); *Water of Kane* (Honolulu: Friends of the Library of Hawaii, 1980), which documents the lives of Japanese contract laborers in the late nineteenth century; and Bushnell's last book, *The Gifts of Civilization: Germs and Genocide in Hawaiʻi* (1993), which historicizes the introduction of diseases and the mass genocide that ensued.

81. Some suggest that the character Dr. Newman is a fictionalized hybrid of several key actors in colonial medicine in Hawaiʻi. See Dominika Ferens, "Queer Ways of Knowing Islands: O. A. Bushnell," in *Ways of Knowing Small Places: Intersections of American Literature and Ethnography since the 1960s* (Wrocław, Poland: Wydawn Uniwersytetu Wrocławskiego, 2010), 93–108.

82. James Michener, *Hawaii: A Novel* (New York: Random House, 2002).

83. Jodi Byrd, *The Transit of Empire: Indigenous Critiques of Colonialism* (Minneapolis: University of Minnesota Press, 2011); Mark Rifkin, *Beyond Settler Time: Temporal Sovereignty and Indigenous Self-Determination* (Minneapolis: University of Minnesota Press, 2017); Iyko Day, *Alien Capital: Asian Racialization and the Logic of Settler Colonial Capitalism* (Durham, N.C.: Duke University Press, 2016).

84. Bushnell, *Gifts of Civilization*.

85. "Hawaiʻi State Archives Celebrates 110 Years," KITV Island Television, October 29, 2016; updated November 14, 2021. https://www.kitv.com/archive/hawaii-state-archives-celebrates-110-years/video_5df21634-a58d-5b8b-8687-aa09741be3e2.html.

86. Lisa Lowe, "History Hesitant," *Social Text* 33, no. 4 (2015): 85–87.

87. Lowe, "History Hesitant," 85.

88. Lowe, 85.

89. Chien-ting Lin's account of *mi-yi* (secret doctors) interrogates the mediation of state power through medical discourse through the surveillance and management of medical modernity via Japanese colonization of Taiwan. Lin details the process of narrating the self-governing subject of medical modernity as "the power effects of knowledge to modulate normative conducts for the 'art of government,'" which for Lin demonstrates precisely how governance of liberal medical subjects attempts to produce "the applicable citizen to effectuate the productive management of life and health." Chien-ting Lin, "Governing 'Secrecy' in Medical Modernity: Knowledge Power and the Mi-Yi Outlaws," *Inter-Asia Cultural Studies* 16, no. 2 (2015): 234.

90. Osorio, *Dismembering Lāhui*.

91. Governor of Hawaii, *Report of the Governor of the Territory of Hawaii to the Secretary of the Interior 1905* (U.S. G.P.O, 1800), 18.

92. Jason Horn, "Archives of Hawaii," *American Archivist* 16, no. 2 (April 1953): 105–14. Horn notes that, after pressure from "Hawaiian leaders," the federal official "finally consented to leaving the records in the Territory on condition that every effort would be made to secure a fireproof building for their preservation" (106–7). An act approved on July 11, 1903, by the territorial legis-

lature appropriated funds ($36,000) to construct the first building, completed on August 23, 1906, and opened the following day. Tracing the secession of archivists leading the project from 1905 to the 1950s, Horn notes: "The original 1906 building was enlarged in 1930, and construction of an annex is scheduled to begin soon. The 1906 building is located in Palace Square in downtown Honolulu, the Territorial capitol. In the center of the square is Iolani Palace, the capital building, formerly the palace of the reigning Hawaiian monarch, and now the office of the Territorial governor" (108). The new building was equally significant as modern preservation solidified the claim to keep the archives in territorial possession: "The plans for the new building provide for the following facilities on the first floor: Administrative offices; index and search rooms; rooms for immigration records and for photographic and microfilm records; a receiving and repair room; and a fumigation chamber. The second floor will be occupied by an air-conditioned fireproof vault for records storage. A flagged balcony will extend along two sides of the building. Funds for equipment will be requested at the next session of the legislature" (108–9). On initial classification: "The first Archivist's plan for segregating and classifying records called for the following headings:

1. Form of government
2. Departments under different governments
3. Bureaus of the departments, and any further subdivisions found necessary
4. Miscellaneous documents not classifiable under the above headings
5. Segregation by years as far as practicable
6. Collecting together all documents relating to any important event in the history of the country so that in looking up such an event or any document bearing on it, all relevant papers would be together so far as possible

After segregating and classifying the records in this manner, Lydecker planned to make a 'summary' index under these different headings to serve as a finding aid" (110). On the second archivist: "Archivist Taylor engaged in more intensive indexing of special subjects than did his predecessor. He also placed increased emphasis on the translation of Hawaiian-language documents into English on the grounds that many of the Hawaiian words and phrases of 75 and more years earlier were becoming unintelligible to the new generation of Hawaiians. Such Hawaiian-language documents, of course, comprise only a fraction of the Archives' holdings, for even under the monarchy the bulk of the government business was recorded in English" (111). On 1940s immigration: "Most of the reference services for private individuals involves efforts to establish United States citizenship, date of birth, and/or date of arrival in the islands. Probably the most-used files in the Archives are the ships' passenger manifests, containing the names of all immigrants to and emigrants from the islands,

1843–1900; and the naturalization records, methodically kept from 1844 to 1900. These records have been extensively indexed to make possible more rapid service. The indexing has been particularly difficult because of the large number of Chinese and Japanese names involved. The records are the only means that many individuals have of proving citizenship or pension rights, and—in the case of many older Orientals—of obtaining permission to visit abroad and return" (112). See also Elizabeth H. Wray, "The Archives of the State of Hawaii," *American Archivist* 23, no. 3 (July 1960): 277–84.

93. Horn, "Archives of Hawaii," 107.

94. Horn, 107.

95. Governor of Hawaii, *Report of the Governor of the Territory of Hawaii to the Secretary of the Interior 1905,* 19.

96. Horn, "Archives of Hawaii," 109–10.

97. "Governor Marks Electronic Records Day with First 'Esigned' Proclamation," News Release, State of Hawaii: Office of Enterprise Technology Services. The creation from this angle was reckoning with national and colonial discourses moving across time and space. The open house also coincided with a project that was in the works for some time, which occasioned the Proclamation in Recognition of Electronic Records Day, issued by the governor of Honolulu. The proclamation sets out to recognize the importance of electronic records in understanding and sharing the history of the state and to acknowledge the roles that government agencies and institutions will play in transforming paper-dependent historical record-keeping to a process that better accommodates the paperless future—one designed to capture the archival traces of electronic ephemera and an effective, efficient, and open state government. Indeed, the proclamation reads: "WHEREAS, the Hawai'i State Archives, the state agency legally mandated to preserve and make accessible the historical records of the State, Territory, Republic and Kingdom of Hawai'i in the public trust since 1905, recognizes the importance and preservation of digital records of permanent value throughout the state." State of Hawaii: Proclamation In Recognition of Electronic Records Day, Office of Enterprise Technology Services. https://ets.hawaii.gov/wp-content/uploads/2016/10/Proclamation_-Electronic-Records-Day-10_10_16.pdf.

2. Memory, Memoir, and the Carville Leprosarium

1. *Federal Aid—Hawaii: Hearings before the Committee on Territories House of Representatives,* 77th Cong. 17 (February 9 and 15, 1932), 1.

2. Neel Ahuja, *Biosecurities: Disease Interventions, Empire, and the Government of Species* (Durham, N.C.: Duke University Press, 2016), 201.

3. *Federal Aid—Hawaii: Hearings before the Committee on Territories House of Representatives,* 77th Cong. 17 (February 9 and 15, 1932) (statements of Victor S. Kaleoaloha Houston and Dr. George Walter McCoy).

4. Houston's mother was Caroline Poor Kahikiola Brickwood. "Victor S.

(Kaleoaloha) Houston: 1876–1959," in *Asian and Pacific Islander Americans in Congress, 1900–2017* (Washington, D.C.: Government Printing Office, 2017), 204–10, https://www.govinfo.gov/content/pkg/GPO-CDOC-108hdoc226/pdf/GPO-CDOC-108hdoc226-2-2-12.pdf.

5. *Federal Aid—Hawaii*, 1. Houston later draws out his rationale on federal prisons and the funding of Kalihi Hospital: "Our thought is based upon this general situation which is found in the United States Code 518, which provides for the admission into State institutions of Federal prisoners, and it says that the Attorney General shall contract with the managers or proper authorities having control of prisoners confined in State or Territorial jails, and so forth, for the imprisonment and subsistence and proper employment of such people, and shall pay the expenses of transformation and confinement, chargeable to the United States. In other words, here we have an institution which is set up and is a going concern, and we have felt that in building up a new one, or in taking this over, a contribution might be made paralleling the situation which we find in the Department of Justice; that is to say, it is not an unheard of method of procedure" (12).

6. *Federal Aid—Hawaii*, 16.

7. *Federal Aid—Hawaii*, 20.

8. *Federal Aid—Hawaii*, 5.

9. *Federal Aid—Hawaii*, 5.

10. *Federal Aid—Hawaii*, 5.

11. *Federal Aid—Hawaii*, 8. See also Dean Itsuji Saranillio, *Unsustainable Empire:* Alternative Histories of Hawai'i (Durham, N.C.: Duke University Press, 2018), 152–62. Saranillio discusses Houston's role in charting racial politics of U.S. annexation and Native Hawaiian consent in 1893, specifically as it relates to statehood debates leading up to 1959.

12. Johnson's efforts to create a "union of the white race" by establishing a "Panaryan association" to keep military supremacy in anticipation of "yellow peril" was the central concern of his congressional speech *The Defense of Alaska: The Union of the White Race and the Problem of Universal Peace.* The speech was based on the writing of Edward Alsworth Ross, American professor of sociology at the University of Wisconsin and early supporter of eugenicist policies, including involuntary sterilization. In *The Defense of Alaska,* for example, Ross wrote in a letter sent with his application to the Panaryan Association Johnson is proposing: "Statesmanship is the art of seeing and providing for coming problems a long time in advance, and, therefore, I regard your endeavor to promote the 'get together' spirit among the leading groups of the white race as statesmanlike. I agree with you that, during most of this century at least, the interests of civilization and the well-being of the laboring classes will best be served by preventing the high-pressure areas in Asia from discharging their surplus population into the regions now held by the white race. I have set forth this idea in a chapter of my book *Changing America,* and also implied it in my

book the *Changing Chinese*. I do not assume the superiority of the Aryans over the Mongolians, but I take my stand on the proposition that the terrible struggle for existence, produced in most parts of Asia by certain elements of their civilization, ought not to be communicated to other lands by great streams of migrant coolies with low standards, ready to work for almost any wage. All the low-pressure countries should protect themselves against the high-pressure countries until these countries, by elevating woman, individualizing their people, and restraining their fecundity, have become low-pressure countries." Johnson follows: "The only means to ward off the crisis, the only means to keep the white race in this country from being swamped in a dusky flood, the only insurance policy that will cost us nothing, is the timely union of the great white nations. . . . It is encouraging to know that in this undertaking we are sure of the whole-hearted cooperation of the most powerful man in Europe, the Emperor of Germany, who, as far back as 1895, long before anyone else thought of the yellow peril, uttered his famous warning: 'Völker Europas, wahret eure höchsten Güter!' (Peoples of Europe, guard your highest interests!)." Albert Johnson, *The Defense of Alaska: The Union of the White Race and the Problem of Universal Peace* (Washington, D.C.: Government Printing Office, 1913), 261. On the significance of the Johnson-Reed Act of 1924, see Mae Ngai, *Impossible Subjects: Illegal Aliens and the Making of Modern America* (Princeton, N.J.: Princeton University Press, 2004).

13. *Federal Aid—Hawaii*, 20. Doctor McCoy attempts to refute the Congress member's search for connections to race, however the questions linking race and disease set the tone for the discussion even as the hearings are discussed as a matter of public health. "There has been a lot of stuff of that, and the general impression is that the islanders of the Pacific are more susceptible than other people in general. Personally, I rather doubt that. For some reason most of us are naturally immune to leprosy and do not get it, and under Hawaiian conditions, given the maximum opportunity for contracting the disease, which is the marital relation, only about 5 per cent of the healthy partners of the marriage in which one is a leper will contract the infections. I have the feeling that, given the same geographical distribution, probably about the same percentage of white people would contract it. I do not think race, per se, makes any essential difference in the rest of acquiring leprosy" (20–21).

14. Neel Ahuja describes "dread life" as the biopolitical discourse that manages fear to "activate other forms of [bodily] transition, shifting the very biological character of national immune ecologies," asking under "what conditions are forms of bodily transition experienced as integrated into the linear, everyday unfolding of life toward death?" Ahuja, *Biosecurities*, 9.

15. Michelle Moran, *Colonizing Leprosy: Imperialism and the Politics of Public Health in the United States* (Chapel Hill: University of North Carolina Press, 2007), 12.

16. Jodi Byrd, *The Transit of Empire*: Indigenous Critiques of Colonialism (Minneapolis: University of Minnesota Press, 2011).

17. Maile Arvin analyzes how Western science has defined Polynesia as, and for, white possession and claims to Oceania. Maile Arvin, *Possessing Polynesians: The Science of Settler Colonial Whiteness in Hawai'i and Oceania* (Durham, N.C.: Duke University Press, 2019). Kerri A. Inglis, *Ma'i Lepera: Disease and Displacement in Nineteenth-Century Hawai'i* (Honolulu: University of Hawai'i Press, 2013); J. Kēhaulani Kauanui, *Hawaiian Blood: Colonialism and the Politics of Sovereignty and Indigeneity* (Durham, N.C.: Duke University Press, 2008); Noenoe K. Silva, *Aloha Betrayed: Native Hawaiian Resistance to American Colonialism* (Durham, N.C.: Duke University Press, 2004).

18. Ahuja, *Biosecurities*; Warwick Anderson, *Colonial Pathologies: American Tropical Medicine, Race, and Hygiene in the Philippines* (Durham, N.C.: Duke University Press, 2006); Warwick Anderson, *The Cultivation of Whiteness: Science, Health, and Racial Destiny in Australia* (Durham, N.C.: Duke University Press, 2006).

19. Moran, *Colonizing Leprosy,* 12.

20. Moran, 12.

21. Anderson, *Colonial Pathologies,* 8. Anderson continues: "Saldívar urges us to look at the borderlands between the United States and Mexico as 'the spaces where the nation begins and ends.' But we should remember that the colonial laboratories of the Philippines, Puerto Rico, and Hawaii also were borderlands, where many 'experts' were experimenting with various national bodies, including their own."

22. Ahuja, *Bio" securities,* 62. The segregation order referred to here is the long-standing 1865 Act to Prevent the Spread of Leprosy, which authorized police power to remove and quarantine suspected infectious people in Hawai'i.

23. Michelle Cliff, *Free Enterprise: A Novel of Mary Ellen Pleasant* (San Francisco: City Lights Press, 2004), 35.

24. Ahuja, *Biosecurities,* 9. Also see Priscilla Wald, *Contagious: Cultures, Carriers, and the Outbreak Narrative* (Durham, N.C.: Duke University Press, 2008).

25. Opal Palmer Adisa and Michelle Cliff, "Journey into Speech—A Writer between Two Worlds: An Interview with Michelle Cliff," *African American Review* 28, no. 2 (Summer 1994): 273.

26. Meryl F. Schwartz and Michelle Cliff, "An Interview with Michelle Cliff," *Contemporary Literature* 34, no. 4 (1993): 598; Adisa and Cliff, "Journey into Speech," 80.

27. Cliff, *Free Enterprise,* 45.

28. Cliff, 16. Situating the novel as pushing up against the "official versions" of history, Cliff writes: "They drew up a constitution for a separate African-American state, and took up arms, beginning their war of independence in

October 1859. And when the smoke cleared the name officially attached to the deed was John Brown. Who has ever heard of Annie Christmas, Mary Shadd, Mary Ellen Pleasant? The official version has been printed, bound, and gagged, resides in schools, libraries, the majority unconscious. Serves the common good. Does not cause trouble. Walks across tapestries, the television screen. Does not give aid and comfort to the enemy. Is the stuff of conversations, colloquia; is substantiated—like the Host—in dissertations. The official version is presented to the people. With friezes of heroes, statues free-standing in vestpocket parks, in full costume on Main Street, on auditorium stages in elementary schools, through two-reelers, in silence—who will forget the *Birth of a Nation*? The official version entertains. Illumines the Great White Way. Is hummed along Tin Pan Alley, by song-pluggers eager for a tip. 'I'd walk a million miles for one of your smiles.' Is barked on the midway at the state fair, alongside the hoochie-koochie girls, the dancing bear. Appears in novels sold for a penny, is serialized in Harper's Monthly, in newspapers where the owner sets his own hot type, inks the rollers, feeds the press, waits on the Pulitzer. Is talked over luncheons at the Rotary, Kiwanis, chambers of commerce. Gets top billing on the vaudeville circuit. The official version is in everybody's mouth. On the lips of the toastmasters, chairwomen of garden clubs, the Gold Dust Twins; cluttering dreams, remembered in prayers. This is what happened; this is how it was" (16–17).

29. Cliff describes the project this way: "[*Free Enterprise* is] also set in the Caribbean. The whole novel is about resistance. It has a Jew from Surinam, a woman who becomes a Maroon, and a freedom fighter, and it talks about the Inquisition and the Expulsion of the Jews in 1942. And then there's a Jamaican woman like myself—but it's not me—who joins forces with abolitionists in this country to fight slavery, leaving behind Jamaica because she thinks it's hopeless to struggle there, so she comes to the United States to become a freedom fighter and ends up in a leper colony in Louisiana. The leper colony is not really a leper colony; it's a colony of political activists who have been incarcerated. They spend their days telling each other their histories. One is a Hawaiian and one is from Tahiti. Then Rachel, the Jew, is there, and Annie who is from Jamaica, and they all sit around telling stories to keep history alive. It's much more diverse than my earlier work. It's a historical novel and it's set primarily in the past, but it's much more diverse than the other novels." Schwartz and Cliff, "Interview with Michelle Cliff," 598.

30. Cliff, *Free Enterprise*, 45.

31. Cliff, 45.

32. Cliff, 46.

33. Mark Rifkin, *Beyond Settler Time: Temporal Sovereignty and Indigenous Self-Determination* (Durham, N.C.: Duke University Press, 2017), 179–92. I look to Rifkin's examination of what he calls "temporal sovereignty"—which takes up conversations about what to do with the problem of sovereignty as a

settler-colonial concept that cannot "translate" Indigenous experience into a settler framework—because it centers questions on unsettling settler times. Rifkin notes, for example: "I want to argue for deferring juridical time—or, more specifically, to argue for the potential value of provisionally suspending the question of how temporal sovereignty . . . could or should be operationalized as part of juridical apparatuses and processes" (180). Rifkin's engagement with Indigenous studies and queer theory presents a useful problematizing of settler/straight national temporalities. "To speak of Indigenous orientations suggests processes of being and becoming that emerge out of everyday life. They arise from, among other things, memory, storying, collective practices, dynamics of maturation and family formation, modes of inhabitation and connections to place, encounters with law and policy in their quotidian effects, histories of dispossession and opposition to it, and engagements with nonhuman entities of various kinds. Such processes generate durable frames of reference that guide perception while being affected, and shifted, by events in the present. These temporalities need not be understood either as antithetical to or as derived from official institutions of governance. Rather, multiple forms of sovereignty can coexist, and acknowledging this multiplicity is part of engaging with the density of Indigenous social formations. Native juridical structures continue to bear the pressure of recognition, of being intelligible to non-native institutions while also being subject to ongoing forms of state regulation, and the kinds of negotiations occurring within and through such institutions may not facilitate engagement with the felt knowledge of Native people(s), including experiences of time" (190–92).

34. See the 2008 special issue of *American Indian Culture and Research Journal,* edited by Andrew Jolivétte, which focused on Hurricanes Katrina and Rita as they affected, unveiled, and highlighted the depth of invisibility of American Indians in Louisiana, particularly in relation to U.S. government policy and the media. *American Indian Culture and Research Journal* 32, no. 2 (2008). Also see Dennis Childs, "The Once and Future Slave Plantation," in *Slaves of the State: Black Incarceration from the Chain Gang to the Penitentiary* (Minneapolis: University of Minnesota Press, 2015), 93–140.

35. I thank museum curator and archivist Elizabeth Schexnyder at the National Hansen's Disease Museum at Carville for her insights and knowledge of the Stanley Stein Archive. The public digital history project New Orleans Historical (https://neworleanshistorical.org) features narratives focusing on walking and driving tours of the National Leprosarium in Carville. This digital project emerged from a collaboration between the History Department at the University of New Orleans and the Communication Department at Tulane University. Accessible online and available as an app to use as a guide, the interactive nine-stop tour gives visitors an overview of the small town and its significance to the national medical narratives of the United States. That story, in essence, is that Carville was and continues to be an important site of medical

triumph over Hansen's disease—one of the most stigmatized communicable diseases across the globe, in spite of its transmission rate remaining low. Carville's official status on the National Park Registry adds to that national story, as does its layered uses and transformational institutional character, as noted above. The virtual tour guide begins, for example, with this overview: "In the 1700s, Europeans settled this area known as Indian Camp and developed a plantation economy along the Mississippi River. Robert Camp, a planter from Virginia, began purchasing land here in the 1820s. He farmed sugarcane and owned about 100 enslaved workers. Camp called his plantation 'Woodlawn,' but the older name for the area, Indian Camp, stuck. The thirty-room mansion behind you, to your right, was built in 1895. The architect, Henry Howard, also designed Nottoway Plantation, which is located across the river." As a medical space, Carville represents many things, but how does it represent its public history, its settler narratives, and its histories of slavery—present and, at the same time, hidden, written over, and erased? Walking the modern medicine landscape accounts for some of it. European settlement in the 1700s quickly transforms into a sugar plantation, the Indian Camp Plantation, made and maintained by Robert Camp. Converted into the Louisiana Leper Home, built out of the former slave quarters, it emerges to become the U.S. National Leprosarium.

36. Mary Ann Sternberg, *Along the River Road: Past and Present on Louisiana's Historic Byway,* 3rd edition (Baton Rouge: Louisiana State University Press, 2013), 187.

37. Sternberg, *Along the River Road,* 188.

38. Tiya Miles, *Tales from the Haunted South: Dark Tourism and Memories of Slavery from the Civil War Era* (Chapel Hill: University of North Carolina Press, 2015).

39. Miles, *Tales from the Haunted South,* 17.

40. Miles, 17–18.

41. Marita Sturken, *Tourists of History: Memory, Kitsch, and Consumerism from Oklahoma City to Ground Zero* (Durham, N.C.: Duke University Press, 2007), 12.

42. Priscilla Wald, *Contagious: Cultures, Carriers, and the Outbreak Narrative* (Durham, N.C.: Duke University Press, 2008), 53. See also Ahuja, *Biosecurities.*

43. Wald, *Contagious,* 53.

44. Stanley Stein, *Alone No Longer: The Story of a Man Who Refused to Be One of the Living Dead!* (New York: Funk & Wagnalls, 1963), 53.

45. Claire Manes, *Out of the Shadow of Leprosy: The Carville Letters and Stories of the Landry Family* (Jackson: University of Mississippi Press, 2013), 8. The "ethnic melting pot" at Carville, notes Manes, "[was] united by the microbes that had invaded their bodies and in some cases made them outcasts from their families and themselves."

46. Stein, *Alone No Longer,* 11.

47. Stein, 11.

48. Sidonie Smith and Julia Watson, *Reading Autobiography: A Guide for Interpreting Life Narratives* (Minneapolis: University of Minnesota Press, 2010), 141. Robert Elliott Burns's 1932 autobiography *I Am a Fugitive from a Georgia Chain Gang!* (Athens: University of Georgia Press, 1997) and the film version *I Am a Fugitive from a Chain Gang*, released in the same year, offer another well-known case. Burns, a World War I veteran, robs a diner and is arrested and sentenced to hard labor. He escapes to Chicago and remakes himself as a successful engineer. When he is found out, however, the question of punishing a successful businessman creates a crisis for the community, and he is pardoned as a contributor to society. The theme of white imprisoned bodies found narrative sway, doing the work of igniting serious debate about the failures of the U.S. legal system for white citizens. As a cultural event, *I Am a Fugitive* engaged a wide U.S. audience by making the story of this chain gang prisoner visible. In a 1932 *Time* magazine article, for example, the author notes that Burns's "arrest aroused national interest, [and] stirred up . . . the question of crime & punishment." The "national interest" in this one prisoner constructs a "model citizen" whose punishment did not seem to fit the crime. Burns escaped the chain gang, bringing a public scrutiny to the penal system not as a form of punishment but as one of criminalization. "States & Cities: Fugitive," *Time,* December 26, 1932.

49. James Kyung-Jin Lee, *Pedagogies of Woundedness: Illness, Memoir, and the Ends of the Model Minority* (Philadelphia: Temple University Press, 2021), 24.

50. Lee, *Pedagogies of Woundedness,* 24.

51. Lee, 24.

52. Lee, 24. Lee develops this by looking to the work of Jane Danielewicz, whose book *Contemporary American Memoirs in Action: How to Do Things with Memoir* (Cham, Switzerland: Palgrave Macmillan, 2018) examines memoir as a genre that enables the creation of a public life and advocacy.

53. Stein, *Alone No Longer,* 55.

54. Benjamin Reiss, *Theaters of Madness: Insane Asylums and Nineteenth-Century American Culture* (Chicago: University of Chicago Press, 2008), 52.

55. Michael Rogin, *Blackface, White Noise: Jewish Immigrants in the Hollywood Melting Pot* (Berkeley: University of California Press, 1996), 15.

56. Hartman, *Scenes of Subjection: Terror, Slavery, and Self-Making in Nineteenth-Century America* (New York: Oxford University Press), 19.

57. George C. Doody, "Leper Heroine," *Wanderer,* August 25, 1949, "Joey File," National Hansen's Disease Museum, Carville, La.

58. Tony Gould, *A Disease Apart: Leprosy in the Modern World* (New York: St. Martin's, 2005), 182.

59. Stein, *Alone No Longer,* 258.

60. Stein, 258.

61. José P. Ramirez Jr., *Squint: My Journey with Leprosy* (Jackson: University Press of Mississippi, 2009), 55.

62. Ramirez, *Squint,* 55.

63. Cheryl Harris, "Whitewashing Race: Scapegoating Culture," in *Whitewashing Race: The Myth of a Colorblind Society* (Oakland: University of California Press, 2006), 908. Harris discusses the editor's analysis of colorblind ideology and use of a black/white (or Black/not-Black) binary as a framework for making visible the maintenance of white supremacy in the United States.

64. Ramirez, *Squint*, 55.

65. Cliff, Free Enterprise, 16-17.

66. Smith and Watson, *Reading Autobiography*, 22. For critical analysis of development in memoir, memory, and novels, see: Lisa Lowe, "Autobiography Out of Empire," in *Intimacies of Four Continents* (Durham, N.C.: Duke University Press, 2015); Grace Hong, *The Ruptures of American Capital: Women of Color Feminism and the Culture of Immigrant Labor* (Minneapolis: University of Minnesota Press, 2006); James Kyung Lee, *Urban Triage: Race and the Fictions of Multiculturalism* (Minneapolis: University of Minnesota Press, 2004); Gayatri Chakravorty Spivak, "Three Women's Texts and Circumfession," in *Postcolonialism & Autobiography: Michelle Cliff, David Dabydeen, Opal Palmer Adisa*, ed. Alfred Hornung and Ernstpeter Ruhe (Amsterdam: Rodopi, 1998), 7.

67. *Federal Aid—Hawaii*, 17.

3. Imagining Medical Archives at Olive View

1. Jill Leovy, "Breathing New Life: Olive View: Opened as a TB Sanitarium in 1920, the Hospital, Now a Modern Facility, Turned 75 This Week," *Los Angeles Times,* October 28, 1995, http://articles.latimes.com/1995-10-28/local/me-62120_1_olive-view.

2. Leovy, "Breathing New Life."

3. *California and Western Medicine* is only one of many journals discussing public health and racialized communities during this time. Other articles published by members of the medical community in California include: Karl L. Schaupp, "Medical Care of Migratory Agricultural Workers: A Story of Accomplishment—Presidential Address," *California and Western Medicine* 60, no. 65 (May 1944); "Health Education Media among California's Mexican-Americans," "Tuberculosis among Chinese," "Negroes in California," "Mexicans and Tuberculosis," and "Tuberculosis Programs among the Mexicans," *California and Western Medicine* 61, no. 2 (August 1944). Selma Calmes, medical staff at Olive View, directed me to the *California Western Medicine* journal and generously shared stories and memories of Olive View.

4. Eric Avila, *Popular Culture in the Age of White Flight: Fear and Fantasy in Suburban Los Angeles* (Berkeley: University of California Press, 2004), 4; Kelly Lytle Hernández, *City of Inmates: Conquest, Rebellion, and the Rise of Human Caging in Los Angeles, 1771–1965* (Chapel Hill: University of North Carolina Press, 2017), 167.

5. "Migratory Agricultural Workers of California: Their Health Care," *California and Western Medicine* 60, no. 2 (1944): 49.

6. "Migratory Agricultural Workers of California," 49.

7. Gilbert G. Gonzalez defines the "Mexican Problem" as "a culture" that relies on a belief that "predisposed Mexicans to laziness and poverty, to a 'Manana syndrome,' a proclivity to violence and heavy drinking, low intellectual abilities and more." Gilbert G. Gonzalez, *Chicano Education in the Era of Segregation* (Dallas: University of North Texas Press, 2013), 5–6. See also Emily K. Abel, *Tuberculosis and the Politics of Exclusion: A History of Public Health and Migration to Los Angeles* (New Brunswick, N.J.: Rutgers University Press, 2007); Lee Bebout, *Whiteness on the Border: Mapping the U.S. Racial Imagination in Brown and White* (New York: NYU Press, 2016); Mike Davis, *City of Quartz: Excavating the Future in Los Angeles* (London: Verso, 2006); Kelly Lytle Hernández, *Migra! A History of the U.S. Border Patrol* (Berkeley: University of California Press, 2010); Natalia Molina, *Fit to Be Citizens? Public Health and Race in Los Angeles, 1879–1939* (Berkeley: University of California Press, 2006); Natalia Molina, *How Race Is Made in America: Immigration, Citizenship, and the Historical Power of Racial Scripts* (Berkeley: University of California Press, 2014).

8. See Tomás Almaguer, *Racial Fault Lines: The Historical Origins of White Supremacy in California* (Berkeley: University of California Press, 1994); Luis Alvarez, *The Power of the Zoot: Youth Culture and Resistance during World War II* (Berkeley: University of California Press, 2008); Ruha Benjamin, *People's Science: Bodies and Rights on the Stem Cell Frontier* (Stanford, Calif.: Stanford University Press, 2013); Nayan Shah, *Contagious Divides: Epidemics and Race in San Francisco's Chinatown* (Berkeley: University of California Press, 2001); Alexandra Minna Stern, *Eugenic Nation: Faults and Frontiers of Better Breeding in Modern America* (Berkeley: University of California Press, 2005); Harriet A. Washington, *Medical Apartheid: The Dark History of Medical Experimentation on Black Americans from Colonial Times to the Present* (New York: Doubleday, 2006).

9. Molina, *How Race Is Made in America*, 100.

10. Stern, *Eugenic Nation*, 102.

11. Benjamin, *People's Science*, 3.

12. See Laurie B. Green, John Raymond McKiernan-González, and Martin Anthony Summers, "Introduction: Making Race, Making Health," in *Precarious Prescriptions: Contested Histories of Race and Health in North America*, ed. Laurie B. Green, John Raymond McKiernan-González, and Martin Anthony Summers (Minneapolis: University of Minnesota Press, 2014), vii–xxviii.

13. David Gutiérrez, *Walls and Mirrors: Mexican Americans, Mexican Immigrants, and the Politics of Ethnicity* (Berkeley: University of California Press, 1995), 91.

14. Vicki L. Ruiz, *Cannery Women, Cannery Lives: Mexican Women, Unionization, and the California Food Processing Industry, 1930–1950* (Albuquerque: University of New Mexico Press, 1987), 7. The conflation of race and disease shaped the ways the state sought to manage the development of the city not

only around a color line but out of the nativism that persisted through narratives of foreignness and noncitizenship. On the framing of community health, diet, and contagious disease in Mexican labor camps and houses, David Gutiérrez notes that of the Mexican families documented (1,668 individuals), over half reported having little or no meat in their regular diet, just under half reported rarely having fresh vegetables, and under half said their children had milk daily. Gutiérrez concludes that "even before the depths of the Great Depression, Mexican Americans and Mexican immigrants in Los Angeles County suffered infant mortality rates that ranged from twice as high as to five times higher than those of the general population." Gutiérrez, *Walls and Mirrors*, 91.

   15. Molina, *Fit to Be Citizens?*, 1.

   16. Abel, *Tuberculosis and the Politics of Exclusion*, 86–87. There were, however, ongoing campaigns to raise funds, and charity organizations such as the Jewish Consumptive Relief Association that ultimately played crucial roles in acquiring funds and shaping the narratives of need, philanthropy, and benevolence.

   17. Molina, *Fit to Be Citizens?*, 143.

   18. For the intersecting ways these discourses surface around race and representation, see Lytle Hernández, *Migra!*; Curtis Marez, *Drug Wars: The Political Economy of Narcotics* (Minneapolis: University of Minnesota Press, 2004).

   19. Molina, *How Race Is Made in America*, 35.

   20. Thomas Dormandy, *The White Death: A History of Tuberculosis* (New York: NYU Press, 2000).

   21. Lisa Lowe argues for understanding "archives of liberalism" as a model for analyzing economies of "affirmation and forgetting" that structures and formalizes in official archives of "liberalism, and liberal ways of understanding." The notion of freedom for "man," as defined by European and North American philosophical frameworks, at the same time relegates others to "geographical and temporal spaces that are constituted as backward, uncivilized, and unfree." The model is particularly important for reading narratives of freedom made possible by forgetting, denying, or erasing colonial slavery, dispossession, and displaced peoples across continents. It problematizes the notion that social inequality is resolvable through rights discourse defined by groups categorized as fully "human," while at the same time locating other subjects, practices, and geographies "at a distance from 'the human.'" Lisa Lowe, *The Intimacies of Four Continents* (Durham, N.C.: Duke University Press, 2015), 3–4.

   22. Lisa Lowe, *Immigrant Acts: An Asian American Cultural Politics* (Durham, N.C.: Duke University Press, 1996), 2.

   23. Alejandro Morales, *The Captain of All These Men of Death* (Tempe, Ariz.: Bilingual Press/Editorial Bilingüe), 1.

   24. Gregory Morales, "The Captain of All These Men of Death: Tuberculosis at the Olive View Sanitarium" (master's thesis, University of California, Los Angeles, 1996).

25. G. Morales, "Captain of All These Men of Death," 16–27.

26. On critical histories of California's twentieth-century Spanish colonial fantasies, see Carey McWilliams, *California: The Great Exception*, rev. ed. (Berkeley: University of California Press, 1999); Carey McWilliams, *North from Mexico: The Spanish-Speaking People of the United States* (Philadelphia: J. B. Lippincott, 1949); Mike Davis, Kelly Mayhew, and Jim Miller, *Under the Perfect Sun: The San Diego Tourists Never See* (New York: New Press, 2005); Charles A. Sepulveda, "Hallucinations of the Spanish Imaginary and the Idealized Hotel California," *California History* 99, no. 3 (2022): 2–24.

27. See Marc García-Martínez, *The Flesh-and-Blood Aesthetics of Alejandro Morales: Disease, Sex, and Figuration* (San Diego: San Diego State University Press, 2014); José Garza, "Social Turbulence as Reflected in Alejandro Morales' Novelistic Techniques" (PhD diss., Indiana University, 2006); José Antonio Palacios Gurpegui, *Alejandro Morales: Fiction Past, Present, Future Perfect* (Tempe, Ariz.: Bilingual Review/Press, 1996); Shimberlee Jirón-King, "Illness, Observation, and Contradiction: Intertext and Intrahistory in Alejandro Morales's *The Captain of All These Men of Death*," *Bilingual Review/La Revista Bilingüe* 29, no. 1 (2008): 3–13; James Kyung-Jin Lee, *Urban Triage: Race and the Fictions of Multiculturalism* (Minneapolis: University of Minnesota Press, 2004), 36–63.

28. Alejandro Morales, *The Captain of All These Men of Death* (Tempe, Ariz.: Bilingual Press/Editorial Bilingüe, 2008), xii. Morales's other novels provide important cues for identifying his theorizations of history through cultural production. His most critically acclaimed novel, *The Brick People* (Houston: Arte Público Press, 1992), for example, fictionalizes generations of Mexican brickmakers and laborers at the Los Angeles Simons Brick Company. The story depicts northern Mexico and California labor and cultural history through the eyes of these workers, yet the engagement with a deep historical archive and his own family's narratives are hauntingly present.

29. Morales, *Captain of All These Men of Death*, 150.

30. Stella Cardwell, "Mission de San Fernando," *Olive View-Point* 12, no. 4 (September 1945), quoted in G. Morales, "Captain of All These Men of Death," 8. Kelly Lytle Hernández describes the Spanish colonial period as "the first experiment in human caging" in Tongva territory. In the 1770s, Spanish settlers used caging to discipline Native rebellion and to control, coerce, and ultimately convert unmarried Tongva women and girls by locking them in dormitories at night. Priests used caging as a method of conversion by forcing thousands of baptisms. As Los Angeles developed, the legal designation of Native peoples as "minors" effectively subjugated the population as wards of the church and state. Lytle Hernández, *City of Inmates*, 25–27.

31. Lawrence Grossberg, "On Postmodernism and Articulation: An Interview with Stuart Hall," in *Stuart Hall: Critical Dialogues in Cultural Studies*, ed. Kuan-Hsing Chen and David Morley (London: Routledge, 1996), 142–43.

32. A. Morales, *Captain of All These Men of Death*, 3.

33. A. Morales, 96.

34. A. Morales, 96–97.

35. G. Morales, "Captain of All These Men of Death," 8.

36. For detailed and systemic techniques developed to enable scientists to perform experiments on prisoners, see Allen M. Hornblum, *Acres of Skin: Human Experiments at Holmesburg Prison—A Story of Abuse and Exploitation in the Name of Medical Science* (New York: Routledge, 1998); Washington, *Medical Apartheid*, 244–70.

37. A. Morales, *Captain of All These Men of Death*, 97. For an analysis of the eugenics movement in the United States and its enduring impact on gender, race, and sexuality, see Nancy Ordover, *American Eugenics: Race, Queer Anatomy, and the Science of Nationalism* (Minneapolis: University of Minnesota Press, 2003).

38. A. Morales, *Captain of All These Men of Death*, 97. This section of the novel depicts multiple examples of violence to tease out the disciplinary nature of the sanatorium, focusing on the racial violence of the Zoot Suit Riots and the mundane and dangerous realities for queer patients.

39. A. Morales, 97. Taken from interviews with the author's uncle, Robert Contreras had several surgeries, including rib removal, at Olive View. His memory of the event, as noted in Gregory Morales's thesis: "When I got the operation, a colored girl went before me. She died, and then I was next. Man, I was nervous. In fact, they gave me steak, a last meal, and the nurse asked me how was it. I didn't taste it. I didn't feel like steak." Contreras interview, February 11, 1996, quoted in G. Morales, "Captain of All These Men of Death," 19.

40. Along with animals (monkeys and guinea pigs), medical facilities developing treatments were testing them in dangerously high doses. Harshini Mukundan and colleagues note that Dapsone was used at Carville Leprosarium in the 1940s, and that Dapsone, at a dose of 100 mg, eventually became the standard treatment for leprosy, but only after six years of experimenting with it at high levels. Alejandro Morales represents the distribution of Dapsone at Olive View at doses of 1,000 and 2,000 mg. See Harshini Mukundan et al., *Tuberculosis, Leprosy, and Other Mycobacterial Diseases of Man and Animals: The Many Hosts of Mycobacteria* (Boston: CABI, 2015), 481. Indeed, Tony Gould notes that, at Carville Leprosarium, "the drug, marketed by the Detroit pharmaceutical firm, Parke-Davis, under the trade name Promin, consisted of glucose sulphone sodium. Sulphone drugs were not new; the compound known as DDS—or diamino diphenyl sulphone, to give its full title—had been synthesised by German chemists as early as 1908, but its bactericidal possibilities had not been considered until the late 1930s. Parke-Davis were happy to provide the drug for free if Dr. Fage wanted to experiment with it at Carville." See Tony Gould, *A Disease Apart* (New York: St. Martin's Press, 2005), 248.

41. A. Morales, *Captain of All These Men of Death*, 222–23.

42. A. Morales, 97.
43. A. Morales, 193.
44. A. Morales, 176.
45. Gurpegui, *Alejandro Morales*, 8.
46. A. Morales, *Captain of All These Men of Death*, 67.
47. A. Morales, 2–3.

Epilogue

1. Cutler's papers were moved from the University of Pittsburgh to the National Archives in Atlanta, Georgia. Digitized versions are available on the National Archives website, CDC, Record Group 442, "Records of Dr. John C. Cutler," https://www.archives.gov/research/health/cdc-cutler-records.

2. For extensive discussion of the dilemmas surrounding historicizing the Tuskegee syphilis experiments and their ongoing historical and cultural traps and pitfalls, see Susan M. Reverby, *Examining Tuskegee: The Infamous Syphilis Study and Its Legacy* (Chapel Hill: University of North Carolina Press, 2009); Susan M. Reverby, *Tuskegee's Truths: Rethinking the Tuskegee Syphilis Study* (Chapel Hill: University of North Carolina Press, 2000).

3. Reverby, *Tuskegee's Truths*, 8.

4. In a 2018 lecture entitled "The Open Secret of Racial Capitalist Violence" (Unit for Criticism & Interpretive Theory, University of Illinois Urbana-Champaign, March 27, 2018), Jodi Melamed points to the "open secret" of administrative logics as working "to reproduce capitalist violence as an open secret by seeking to operationalize what the human can mean for capitalism . . . through repertoires of rights and race; to operationalize land or territoriality for capital circulations, often through colonial routines; and to repress what it represents as disorder through capitalist making and capitalist preserving violence done by agents of law and order."

Among the many scholars who interrogate the sophistication and complexity through which the institution of medicine manages knowledge, Harriet A. Washington's account of researching the medical archive in search of medical experimentation on Black Americans in *Medical Apartheid* is one of the more telling. For centuries, conversations and racist practices have operated with little scrutiny, understanding medicine's role in the public eye as humanitarian, working for the public good, and therefore largely unconcerned with justifying its methods and practices beyond the approval of the scientific community. Washington suggests that, in addition to the physical inaccessibility to medical research, generally housed in universities not for a general public, the impenetrable scientific language obscures acts and behavior that would otherwise be classified as violence, harmful, and dangerous: "It is medical researchers themselves who have documented the proof of this long, unhappy history of African Americans as research subjects. Even so, this history has been a challenge to document because it has been hidden in plain sight—widely scattered, distorted, and rendered all but unrecognizable as abuse by heavy editorializing. As I recall the years I have spent ferreting out these experiments bit by bit, examining their patterns, and probing the mind-sets that they revealed, I am put in mind of the legal discovery process. A favored ploy is to provide the opposing side with all the information it seeks—buried in towering mountains of unrelated or tangentially related documents. . . . Generalized professional journals such as the *Journal of the American Medical Association* and the *New England Journal of Medicine* are not available in bookstores or on newsstands. Specialized medical journals are even less accessible, and access was even more restricted in past decades. The medical libraries that house these journals have historically been closed to the public and most remain so; indeed, I have been challenged while entering such libraries while a student or instructor at various northern universities. Moreover, physical access to such journals would constitute only the first hurdle: The medical jargon in which such research papers are couched is often impenetrable even to well-educated nonmedical people." Harriet A. Washington, *Medical Apartheid: The Dark History of Medical Experimentation on Black Americans from Colonial Times to the Present* (New York: Penguin Books, 2008), 12–13.

See also Ruha Benjamin, *People's Science: Bodies and Rights on the Stem Cell Frontier* (Stanford, Calif.: Stanford University Press, 2013); Alexandra Minna Stern, *Eugenic Nation: Faults and Frontiers of Better Breeding in Modern America* (Minneapolis: University of Minnesota Press, 2005); Dorothy Roberts, *Killing the Black Body: Race, Reproduction, and the Meaning of Liberty* (New York: Knopf Doubleday, 1998).

5. The "Joint Statement by Secretaries Clinton and Sebelius on a 1946–1948 Study" was published in English and in Spanish and distributed widely to the media in 2010.

6. U.S. Department of Health and Human Services, Secretaries Hilary Clinton and Kathleen Sebelius, "Joint Statement by Secretaries Clinton and Sebelius on a 1946–1948 Study," October 1, 2010. https://2009-2017.state.gov/secretary/20092013clinton/rm/2010/10/148464.htm.

7. Presidential Commission for the Study of Bioethical Issues, *Ethically Impossible: STD Research in Guatemala from 1946 to 1948*, Washington D.C., September 2011, 3.

8. While much of this discussion intentionally began as an official public statement, archived by the Bioethics Commission and housed by HHS government websites, the online documents have largely been removed. The Bioethics Commission archive (formerly www.bioethics.gov) is now hosted by Georgetown University (Presidential Commission for the Study of Bioethical Issues, https://bioethicsarchive.georgetown.edu/pcsbi/). References to the Guatemala experiments on government websites have been removed.

9. Cutler went on to become the assistant surgeon general in 1958 and later served as professor and dean of the Graduate School of Public Health at the University of Pittsburgh until the 1990s. The University of Pittsburgh accepted his personal and professional papers, which were held unnoticed until 2010. See also Susan M. Reverby, "'Normal Exposure' and Inoculation Syphilis: A PHS 'Tuskegee' Doctor in Guatemala, 1946–1948," *Journal of Policy History* 23, no. 1 (2011): 9–12.

10. Reverby, *Examining Tuskegee*, 146–47. "Syphilis's transfer through injection in an experiment also requires techniques that have to be done quickly. When this was done on prisoners at Sing Sing Penitentiary in New York in the mid-1950s, an infected rabbit was killed, its testes were ground up, and the bacteria were injected into the 62 subjects within two hours. This usually produced a nodule that became ulcerated at the point of the injection. The inoculum in the Sing Sing study had to be made at 2,000 times the normal infection level to make sure the prisoners got syphilis" (201).

11. Scholars discuss the discursive chasm between the narrative of a rogue scientist doing harm, on one side, and the structural violence that has always been at the heart of medical science, on the other side. See Harriet Washington's comprehensive study, *Medical Apartheid*.

12. Jim Handy, *Revolution in the Countryside: Rural Conflict and Agrarian Reform in Guatemala, 1944–1954* (Chapel Hill: University of North Carolina Press, 1994), 8–9.

13. Quoted in Presidential Commission for the Study of Bioethical Issues, *Ethically Impossible*, 74; John Cutler, Final Syphilis Report, February 24, 1955, PCSBI HSPI Archives, CTLR_0000655.

14. Presidential Commission for the Study of Bioethical Issues, *Ethically Impossible*, 74; G. Robert Coatney to John Cutler, May 17, 1947, PCSBI HSPI Archives, CTLR_0001122.

15. "Letter from Roberto Robles Chinchilla to John Cutler," in Presidential Commission for the Study of Bioethical Issues, *Ethically Impossible*, 35.

16. Donald G. McNeil Jr., "U.S. Apologizes for Syphilis Tests in Guatemala," *New York Times*, October 1, 2010, https://www.nytimes.com/2010/10/02/health/research/02infect.html.

17. McNeil, "U.S. Apologizes for Syphilis Tests in Guatemala."

18. Presidential Commission for the Study of Bioethical Issues, *Ethically Impossible*, vi, emphasis added.

19. Sushma Subramanian, "Worse Than Tuskegee," Slate, February 26, 2017, www.slate.com/articles/health_and_science/cover_story/2017/02/guatemala_syphilis_experiments_worse_than_tuskegee.html.

20. Johns Hopkins University's public relations campaign website, which documents their responses and refusal to acknowledge their involvement with the case, is currently available here: "U.S. Government Study in 1940s

Guatemala," Johns Hopkins Medicine, https://www.hopkinsmedicine.org/guatemala_study/index.html.

A Letter to the Johns Hopkins Community—April 1, 2015
SUBJECT: Challenges from the past

Dear Member of the Johns Hopkins Community,

More than 60 years ago, the U.S. government conducted an unconscionable and unethical experiment in Guatemala, in which U.S. government researchers deliberately infected vulnerable citizens of Guatemala with syphilis and other infectious diseases. We feel profound sympathy for the individuals and families impacted by this deplorable study.

When the details of this study came to light, a Presidential Commission determined that the Guatemala Study was funded and conducted by the United States government. In 2010, the President of the United States, the Secretary of State and the Secretary of Health and Human Services apologized to all affected. In 2012, a federal district court concluded that the pleas of victims for relief are more appropriately directed to the political branches of the federal government.

Today, attorneys representing Guatemalan plaintiffs announced that they are suing The Johns Hopkins University and Johns Hopkins Health System, alleging that Johns Hopkins was responsible for the study. The plaintiffs' essential claim in this case is that prominent Johns Hopkins faculty members' participation on a government committee that reviewed funding applications was tantamount to conducting the research itself, and therefore that Johns Hopkins should be held liable.

Neither assertion is true.

This was not a Johns Hopkins study. Johns Hopkins did not initiate, pay for, direct or conduct the study in Guatemala. Participation in the review of government research was then and is today separate from being a Johns Hopkins employee, and no nonprofit university or hospital has ever been held liable for a study conducted by the U.S. government.

As a leading global research university, Johns Hopkins values rigorous and open scrutiny of history, even when it is complex and uncomfortable.

We know that historians have previously linked prominent Johns Hopkins faculty members in various ways to other unethical government research studies in Tuskegee and Terre Haute. Although separate from the Guatemala lawsuit, these studies were all deplorable and all demand reflection upon the broader legacy of unethical research. It is important to confront and learn from the past. At the same time, we cannot let unfounded allegations go unchallenged. We will defend the institution vigorously in court against legal responsibility for the government's Guatemala study.

If you would like more information about the university's position on the lawsuit, we have released a media statement that you can find here [link removed], along with information about the Presidential Commission on the research in Guatemala and its findings.

Sincerely,

Ronald J. Daniels
President, The Johns Hopkins University

Paul B. Rothman, M.D.
Dean of the Medical Faculty
CEO, Johns Hopkins Medicine

Michael J. Klag, M.D., M.P.H.
Dean, Johns Hopkins Bloomberg School of Public Health

21. Walter Benjamin, "Critique of Violence," in *Reflections: Essays, Aphorisms, Autobiographical Writings* (San Diego: Harcourt Brace Jovanovich, 1978).

22. Tom Rivers, *Tom Rivers: Reflections on a Life in Medicine and Science* (Cambridge, Mass.: MIT Press, 1967); Reverby, "'Normal Exposure' and Inoculation Syphilis."

23. Marita Sturken, *Untangled Memories: The Vietnam War, the AIDS Epidemic, and the Politics of Remembering* (Berkeley: University of California Press, 1997), 259.

INDEX